ACLS Quick Review
Study Guide

Barbara Aehlert, RN

Director, EMS Education and Research
Samaritan Health System
Phoenix, Arizona

with 91 illustrations

Illustrations (except ECGs and those otherwise noted) by
Kimberly Battista

Publisher: David T. Culverwell
Executive Editor: Richard A. Weimer
Developmental Editor: Julie Scardiglia
Book Design and Production: Cynthia Edmiston

Printed in the United States of America

Mosby-Year Book, Inc.
11830 Westline Industrial Drive
St. Louis, MO 63146

PREFACE

This book is designed for use by physicians, nurses, prehospital providers, respiratory therapists and allied health professionals preparing for the American Heart Association Advanced Cardiac Life Support (ACLS) Provider Course.

Many hospitals with critical care areas require their physician, nursing and respiratory therapy staffs to participate in, and successfully complete, the AHA ACLS Provider course. ACLS courses, whether the conventional two-day or extended (over a period of weeks) format, cover a considerable amount of information in a short period. This book is designed to supplement the AHA materials and provides a summary of the fundamental concepts presented in the ACLS course based on the American Heart Association guidelines printed in the October 28, 1992 JAMA.

Since publication of the October 28, 1992 JAMA, the National AHA ACLS Subcomittee has met to review and clarify questions that have arisen since publication of the new guidelines. The material contained in this text covers the latest information available, including changes discussed by the National AHA Subcommittee.

The American Heart Association has identified the following areas as "core" material to be taught in the ACLS Course:

Myocardial Infarction

Airway Adjuncts and Endotracheal Intubation

Dysrhythmia Recognition and therapy, including algorithms

Electrical Therapy

Intravenous Techniques

Cardiovascular Pharmacology

Special Resuscitation Situations

Those areas evaluated in the ACLS Provider course include:

Airway Adjuncts and Intubation

Dysrhythmia Recognition and Therapy

Megacode including:

    Sole-rescuer basic life support skills

    Defibrillation

    Endotracheal intubation

    Intravenous medications

Written evaluation

The chapters in this text are consistent with those identified as "core" material and provide instructional objectives followed by a review of the critical elements related to the subject.

A pretest, post-test and additional quizzes with answer sheets are provided for self-evaluation. Answer keys for each test and quiz are provided with explanations and references, when possible, to the 1992 JAMA.

This text is designed to assist you in preparing for the ACLS course, as an adjunct to the lectures and skills sessions provided during the course, and as a reference upon completion of the course. I hope you find this text of assistance and welcome your comments and suggestions.

Barbara Aehlert, R.N.

DEDICATION

To Dean, Andrea and Sherri

ACKNOWLEDGMENTS

I would like to thank:

Those who have attended ACLS courses in which I have taught. Your questions provide me with an endless opportunity to learn and grow and have taught me more than any formal course of instruction ever could.

Mary Alice Witzel, R.N. and **Marcia Barry, R.N., MSN,** two very dear and extraordinary friends who offer encouragement, advice and a willing ear whenever I need it. I sincerely appreciate your support and cherish our friendship.

Debby Sorensen, R.N. a very dear friend and outstanding clinical nurse who contributed many of the rhythm strips used in this text.

Kathryn M. Lewis, R.N., Ph.D., an exceptional educator who taught my first EKG class and from whom I have learned so very much over the years.

Angie Golden, R.N., William Loughran, R.N. and **Julie Sweeney, R.N.,** who provided an objective evaluation of my first efforts with this project and never fail to provide an opportunity for stimulating discussions on any topic.

Robert Baron, M.D., Lester Tukan, M.D., Todd Taylor, M.D., David Streitwieser, M.D., John Gallagher, III, M.D., John Raife, M.D. and **Peter Vann, M.D.,** who have graciously shared their thoughts regarding the management of patients in many interesting discussions over the years.

Fred Hosler, M.D. and **Shirley Hosler, R.N.** A special thanks to Fred, for the many hours spent patiently answering my never-ending questions.

Peggy Gladys-Dehm, R.N., with whom I have enjoyed discussing methods of teaching ACLS and from whom I have learned much in the process.

Richard Weimer and **Julie Scardiglia** of Mosby Lifeline whose patience and encouragement made this undertaking possible. A special thanks to Julie whose humor, delightful personality and expertise made this project fun and exciting.

Cynthia Edmiston of Merrifield Graphics & Publishing Service, Inc., who patiently and painstakingly made the necessary changes to this material.

My family, for their patience during the long hours spent at the computer drafting, revising and perfecting this book. Thanks Dean, Andrea, Sherri, Mom, Ernie, Kathy, Doug, Steve and Dad for your love and support.

A very special thanks to my husband Dean. Your love, encouragement, advice and support have kept me going while I pursued this project.

Barbara Aehlert, R.N.

CONTENTS

Pretest

1. Endotracheal intubation:

   a. is contraindicated in unresponsive patients
   b. eliminates the risk of aspiration of gastric contents
   c. should be preceded by efforts to ventilate by another method
   d. when attempted, should be performed in less than 60 seconds

2. A 78 year old male is in cardiac arrest. CPR is in progress and an IV line has not yet been established. The sites of first choice for cannulation while chest compressions are being performed are:

   a. the subclavian or antecubital vein
   b. the internal or external jugular vein
   c. the femoral or internal jugular vein
   d. the antecubital or external jugular vein

3. The most common cause of pulseless electrical activity is:

   a. hypoxia
   b. acidosis
   c. hypovolemia
   d. hyperkalemia

4. A 45 year old male is complaining of chest pain radiating to the neck and left arm. His blood pressure is 124/78, respiratory rate 16. The cardiac monitor displays the following rhythm. Management of this patient should include:

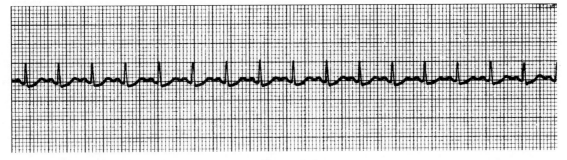

Figure 1-1

   a. administer atropine 1.0 mg IV bolus
   b. administer adenosine, 6 mg, rapid IV bolus
   c. administer supplemental oxygen, monitor the patient for dysrhythmias and administer medications for relief of pain
   d. monitor the patient for dysrhythmias, administer supplemental oxygen and administer prophylactic lidocaine

5. Hypotension as a result of verapamil administration may be treated with the use of which of the following medications?

   a. isoproterenol
   b. atropine sulfate
   c. calcium chloride
   d. bretylium tosylate

6. If the initial systolic blood pressure is less than 90-100 mm Hg in patients with acute pulmonary edema, an infusion of which of the following should be initiated?

   a. lidocaine
   b. dopamine
   c. dobutamine
   d. sodium nitroprusside

7. A 63 year old male is admitted with an acute inferior wall myocardial infarction. He is presently on oxygen at four liters/minute by nasal cannula and has an IV infusing at a TKO rate. As you begin your assessment of this patient, you note a change in his rhythm on the cardiac monitor. His blood pressure is 118/66, respirations 18. The patient is awake, alert and responsive and denies chest pain or dyspnea. The monitor shows ventricular tachycardia at a rate of 170/minute. What action should you take at this time?

   a. check the patient's carotid pulse for 3 minutes
   b. confirm the rhythm in another lead and initiate CPR
   c. administer 2.5 mg of verapamil slow IV push over 2-3 minutes
   d. administer 1-1.5 mg/kg of lidocaine IV bolus and reassess the patient

8. The most important consequence of prolonged underwater submersion without ventilation is hypoxemia.

   a. true
   b. false

9. The correct dose of epinephrine, when administered through an endotracheal tube is:

   a. 0.5 mg
   b. 1.0 mg
   c. 2-2.5 mg
   d. 1-1.5 mg/kg

10. A 66 year old male is complaining of palpitations. He denies chest pain or difficulty breathing. His blood pressure is 136/84, respiratory rate is 16. Breath sounds are clear bilaterally. The patient is awake, alert and his skin is warm and dry. The cardiac monitor shows ventricular tachycardia at 196 beats/minute. Initial antidysrhythmic therapy with lidocaine and procainamide have proven ineffective. The patient's condition remains unchanged. As you prepare to administer bretylium to this patient, you recall that in this situation bretylium should be administered according to which of the following recommended guidelines?

    a. 5-10 mg/kg IV infusion over 8-10 minutes
    b. 1.5 mg/kg IV bolus, repeated in 20 minutes
    c. 20 mg/min IV infusion, to a total of 1.2 grams
    d. 5 mg/kg rapid IV bolus and repeated in 8-10 minutes with 10 mg/kg

11. Lidocaine:

    a. is a potent arterial vasodilator
    b. is administered as a 1-1.5 mg/kg bolus in VF
    c. is administered via continuous IV infusion in VF
    d. should be administered prophylactically in uncomplicated acute MI or ischemia without ventricular ectopy

12. Endotracheal intubation:

    1. Reduces the risk of aspiration
    2. Should be performed before defibrillation for the patient in VF
    3. Provides a route for administration of some medications
    4. Should not be attempted by inexperienced professionals

    a. 1, 2
    b. 2, 3
    c. 1, 2, 4
    d. 1, 3, 4

13. Which of the following is NOT an effect of isoproterenol administration?

    a. increased heart rate
    b. increased force of myocardial contraction
    c. causes significant peripheral vasoconstriction
    d. may precipitate ventricular ectopy due to increased myocardial work load

14. An 86 year old female is in cardiac arrest. The cardiac monitor shows ventricular fibrillation. Your best course of action will be to:

    a. charge the defibrillator to 50J and prepare to defibrillate
    b. perform CPR until a defibrillator is available and then defibrillate with 200J
    c. intubate the patient, establish an IV of 5% dextrose in water and defibrillate with 200J
    d. perform CPR until a defibrillator is available, turn on the synchronizer switch and charge the paddles to 200J

15. Verapamil:

    a. is an α-adrenergic stimulating agent
    b. is useful in treating symptomatic sinus bradycardia
    c. slows conduction and increases refractoriness in the AV node
    d. is a first-line agent in the management of ventricular tachycardia

16. Adenosine may be of benefit in the treatment of:

    a. pulmonary edema
    b. calcium overdose
    c. profound bradycardia
    d. paroxysmal supraventricular tachycardia

17. Dopamine infusions at 5 mcg/kg/min will likely produce:

    a. peripheral vasoconstriction and marked tachycardia
    b. systemic vasoconstriction and increased renal perfusion
    c. renal blood vessel dilation and peripheral vasoconstriction
    d. β-adrenergic receptor stimulating effects resulting in increased cardiac output

18. Emergent pacing is indicated in all of the following situations EXCEPT:

    a. ventricular fibrillation
    b. hemodynamically compromising bradycardias
    c. bradycardia with malignant escape rhythms unresponsive to pharmacologic therapy
    d. overdrive pacing of refractory tachycardia refractory to pharmacologic therapy or countershock

19. A 56 year old male is complaining his "heart is racing." He is disoriented and having difficulty breathing. Examination reveals a blood pressure of 64/P; a weak, rapid carotid pulse and pale, cool skin. Your ECG shows a narrow-QRS tachycardia at 220 beats/minute. Initial management of this patient should include:

    a. IV administration of 2.5 mg of verapamil
    b. administer sedation, then deliver synchronized countershock at 50 joules
    c. administer sedation, then deliver unsynchronized countershock at 100 joules
    d. reassess the patient's pulse, reconfirm the rhythm on the monitor and then proceed immediately with unsynchronized countershock at 200 joules

20. Which of the following is a non-modifiable risk factor?

    a. obesity
    b. heredity
    c. lack of exercise
    d. cigarette smoking

21. Which of the following statements regarding myocardial infarction is INCORRECT?

    a. 45% of all heart attacks occur in people under age 65
    b. the most common complication of myocardial infarction is cardiac dysrhythmias
    c. aspirin is of no value in improving mortality when used within 24 hours of onset of chest pain
    d. thrombolytic therapy is of greatest benefit if given as soon as possible after onset of symptoms

22. Which of the following factors reduces transthoracic resistance and enhances the chance for successful defibrillation?

    a. the use of lower energy levels (50-75 joules)
    b. single countershocks delivered several minutes apart
    c. administration of sodium bicarbonate before each defibrillation attempt
    d. application of firm pressure (approximately 25 pounds) to conventional defibrillator paddles

23. Management of pulseless electrical activity includes:

    1. Evaluation of breath sounds
    2. Administration of a 1.5 mg/kg lidocaine bolus
    3. Establishing an IV of normal saline or Lactated Ringer's solution
    4. Administration of epinephrine

    a. 1, 2
    b. 2, 3
    c. 1, 4
    d. 1, 3, 4

24. The most prominent medical emergency in the United States today is:

    a. drowning
    b. hypothermia
    c. drug intoxication
    d. sudden death related to coronary artery disease

25. Dopamine, an effective agent for the treatment of hypotension and cardiogenic shock, stimulates alpha, beta and dopaminergic receptors.

    a. true
    b. false

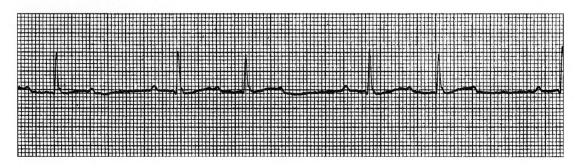

Figure 1-2

26. The rhythm displayed above is:

    a. sinus arrhythmia
    b. first-degree AV block
    c. second degree AV block, Type I
    d. complete (third-degree) AV block

27. Which of the following statements regarding vagal maneuvers is INCORRECT?

    a. carotid sinus pressure should be avoided in older patients
    b. carotid sinus pressure should be avoided if carotid bruits are present
    c. an ECG monitor should be used when carotid sinus pressure is performed
    d. simultaneous bilateral carotid pressure is applied to assure slowing of conduction through the AV node

28. Endpoints of procainamide administration include all of the following EXCEPT:

    a. suppression of the dysrhythmia
    b. respiratory depression develops
    c. a maximum of 17 mg/kg has been administered
    d. the QRS complex widens more than 50% of its original width

29. The correct energy sequence for delivery in the unstable patient in (monomorphic) ventricular tachy-cardia with a pulse would be:

    a. 75-100, 200, 360 joules
    b. 200, 200-300, 360 joules
    c. 100, 200, 300, 360 joules
    d. 50, 100, 200, 300, 360 joules

30. In the management of a symptomatic, narrow-QRS bradycardia, if the maximum dose of atropine had been administered and a pacemaker was not immediately available, your next course of action would include:

    a. lidocaine 1-1.5 mg/kg, IV bolus
    b. procainamide infusion, 20 mg/min
    c. dopamine infusion 5-20 μg/kg/min
    d. isoproterenol infusion, 2-10 μg/min

31. The oropharyngeal airway (OPA):

    1. can only be used in spontaneously breathing patients
    2. is usually well tolerated in the conscious or semiconscious patient
    3. should be used when possible for unconscious patients who are not intubated
    4. may result in airway obstruction if improperly inserted

    a. 1, 2
    b. 3, 4
    c. 1, 2, 3
    d. 1, 3, 4

32. An advantage of central venous access over the peripheral route is:

    a. easier to learn
    b. results in fewer complications
    c. does not require interruption of CPR
    d. more rapid arrival of medications at their sites of action

33. With an oxygen flow rate of 1-6 liters/minute, a nasal cannula can deliver an estimated oxygen con-centration of:

    a. 17-21%
    b. 25-45%
    c. 40-60%
    d. 60-100%

34. The first drug and dosage administered in wide complex tachycardia of uncertain origin is:

    a. adenosine 6 mg IV bolus
    b. atropine 0.5-1.0 mg IV bolus
    c. verapamil 2.5-5.0 mg IV bolus
    d. lidocaine 1-1.5 mg/kg IV bolus

35. A 43 year old female is complaining of chest pain that began approximately 40 minutes ago. Her blood pressure is 76/P, respirations 32 and shallow. Your monitor shows a narrow-QRS tachycardia at 180/minute. The patient is profusely diaphoretic, cool and pale and is losing consciousness. A palpable pulse is present. Recommended treatment for this patient includes:

    a. bretylium 5 mg/kg IV bolus
    b. verapamil 2.5 mg slow IV push
    c. synchronized countershock at 50J
    d. unsynchronized countershock at 100J

36. A 57 year old male is complaining of chest pain and dizziness. His blood pressure is 118/64, respiratory rate 24. The cardiac monitor displays sporadic episodes of Torsades de Pointes. Which of the following treatment measures should be avoided in the management of this patient?

    a. administration of procainamide
    b. administration of magnesium sulfate
    c. consideration of an isoproterenol infusion
    d. defibrillation for any sustained episodes of torsades

37. Which of the following statements regarding norepinephrine is INCORRECT?

    a. norepinephrine usually induces renal and mesenteric vasoconstriction
    b. the efficacy of norepinephrine is reduced if mixed in the same intravenous line as an alkaline solution
    c. norepinephrine decreases myocardial oxygen demand and should be considered early in the management of patients with ischemic heart disease
    d. ischemic necrosis and sloughing of superficial tissues may result from extravasation of norepinephrine

38. First-line medications administered in the management of acute pulmonary edema without hypotension include:

    a. amrinone, aminophylline, digoxin
    b. aspirin, dobutamine, streptokinase
    c. nitroglycerin, nitroprusside, dopamine
    d. furosemide and sublingual nitroglycerin

39. Dobutamine:

    a. stimulates dopaminergic receptors
    b. frequently induces reflex peripheral vasoconstriction
    c. is a synthetic catecholamine useful in the treatment of heart failure
    d. has predominant α-adrenergic receptor stimulating effects that increase myocardial contractility

40. A 65 year old male is in cardiac arrest. The ECG monitor initially showed VF. Defibrillation was promptly administered with sequential unsynchronized countershocks at 200, 300 and 360 joules The patient was successfully intubated and an intravenous line initiated. 1 mg of 1:10,000 epinephrine was administered IV bolus. After circulating the drug with CPR, defibrillation was again performed at 360 joules. The monitor now shows a sinus rhythm at 86 beats/minute with frequent R on T PVCs and runs of VT. A weak pulse is present, there are no spontaneous respirations and the blood pressure is presently 86/54. You should now:

    a. continue CPR until the patient's blood pressure is at least 100 systolic
    b. continue ventilation with a bag-valve device and 100% oxygen, administer a lidocaine bolus and reassess the patient
    c. continue ventilation with a bag-valve device and 100% oxygen, administer 2.5 mg of verapamil and reassess the patient
    d. continue ventilation with a bag-valve device and 100% oxygen, administer 0.5-1.0 mg of atropine and prepare for transcutaneous pacing

41. Which of the following is NOT a desirable feature of a bag-valve device?

    a. non-rebreathing valve
    b. compressible, self-refilling bag
    c. pop-off (pressure release) valve
    d. availability in adult and pediatric sizes

42. Lidocaine may be LETHAL if administered for which of the following rhythms?

    a. ventricular tachycardia
    b. idioventricular (ventricular escape) rhythm
    c. wide complex tachycardia of uncertain origin
    d. sinus tachycardia with premature ventricular complexes

43. Verapamil:

    1. is the drug of choice in wide complex tachycardia of uncertain origin
    2. should be administered over 3-4 minutes when the patient's blood pressure is within the lower range of normal
    3. increases the ventricular fibrillation threshold
    4. should be used with caution in patients who receive long-term β-blocker therapy

    a. 1, 2
    b. 3, 4
    c. 2, 4
    d. 1, 3

44. Advanced cardiac life support medications that may be administered via the endotracheal tube include:

    a. lidocaine, epinephrine, atropine
    b. lidocaine, furosemide, bretylium
    c. lidocaine, atropine, sodium bicarbonate
    d. epinephrine, sodium bicarbonate, calcium chloride

45. Which of the following statements regarding management of the suspected stroke patient is INCORRECT?

    a. lorazepam or diazepam may be used to treat active seizures
    b. 5% dextrose in water is the preferred intravenous solution for administration to the suspected stroke patient
    c. if the patient develops signs of herniation, intubation with hyperventilation may provide a temporary means of reducing increased intracranial pressure
    d. signs and symptoms of acute stroke include an intense or unusually severe headache of sudden onset, aphasia, incoordination and weakness

46. A therapeutic option that is "not indicated, may be harmful" is categorized as:

    a. Class I
    b. Class IIa
    c. Class IIb
    d. Class III

47. Atropine:

1. is the drug of choice in cardiac arrest
2. is the drug of choice for paroxysmal supraventricular tachydysrhythmias
3. may be helpful in pulseless electrical activity and asystolic cardiac arrest
4. may be helpful in symptomatic sinus bradycardia and AV block at the nodal level

a. 1, 2
b. 3, 4
c. 2, 3
d. 1, 4

48. The term "unsynchronized countershock" is synonymous with defibrillation.

a. true
b. false

49. The absolute refractory period:

a. begins with the onset of the P wave and terminates with the end of the QRS complex
b. begins with the onset of the QRS complex and terminates with the end of the T wave
c. begins with the onset of the QRS complex and terminates at approximately the apex of the T wave
d. begins with the onset of the P wave and terminates with the beginning of the QRS complex

50. When sodium bicarbonate is used, 1 mEq/kg should be given as the initial dose, then half this dose every 5 minutes thereafter.

a. true
b. false

PRETEST ANSWER SHEET

1. A   B   C   D
2. A   B   C   D
3. A   B   C   D
4. A   B   C   D
5. A   B   C   D
6. A   B   C   D
7. A   B   C   D
8. A   B   C   D
9. A   B   C   D
10. A   B   C   D
11. A   B   C   D
12. A   B   C   D
13. A   B   C   D
14. A   B   C   D
15. A   B   C   D
16. A   B   C   D
17. A   B   C   D
18. A   B   C   D
19. A   B   C   D
20. A   B   C   D
21. A   B   C   D
22. A   B   C   D
23. A   B   C   D
24. A   B   C   D
25. A   B   C   D

26. A   B   C   D
27. A   B   C   D
28. A   B   C   D
29. A   B   C   D
30. A   B   C   D
31. A   B   C   D
32. A   B   C   D
33. A   B   C   D
34. A   B   C   D
35. A   B   C   D
36. A   B   C   D
37. A   B   C   D
38. A   B   C   D
39. A   B   C   D
40. A   B   C   D
41. A   B   C   D
42. A   B   C   D
43. A   B   C   D
44. A   B   C   D
45. A   B   C   D
46. A   B   C   D
47. A   B   C   D
48. A   B   C   D
49. A   B   C   D
50. A   B   C   D

PRETEST ANSWERS

QUESTION	ANSWER	RATIONALE	JAMA PAGE REFERENCE
1	C	Endotracheal (ET) intubation should be preceded by attempts to ventilate by another method. Endotracheal intubation is indicated in situations where the patient is unable to protect his/her own airway. ET intubation reduces but does not eliminate the risk of aspiration of gastric contents and, when attempted, should be performed in less than 30 seconds.	2201
2	D	If no IV line exists at the time of arrest, the antecubital or external jugular vein should be cannulated first since CPR often has to be interrupted to establish central venous access.	2205
3	C	The most common cause of pulseless electrical activity is hypovolemia.	2219
4	C	All patients suspected of experiencing an MI should be given supplemental oxygen. The rhythm shown is sinus tachycardia without ectopy. Prophylactic lidocaine is no longer recommended. The patient has a good blood pressure and should receive medication for pain relief as soon as possible.	2230
5	C	Calcium chloride (2-4 mg/kg) may be administered for verapamil (a calcium channel blocker) induced hypotension.	2209, 2225
6	B	Dopamine is recommended for hypotension (systolic BP < 90-100) associated with acute pulmonary edema. Norepinephrine is recommended for severe hypotension (systolic BP< 70 mm Hg).	2229
7	D	This patient is clinically stable. Administer 1-1.5 mg/kg of lidocaine IV bolus and reassess.	2223, 2225
8	A	This statement is true.	2246

9	C	The recommended dose of epinephrine, when administered via the endotracheal tube, is 2-2$\frac{1}{2}$ times the IV dose which should be diluted in 10 ml of normal saline or distilled water.	2205
10	A	Bretylium is administered to the patient with a pulse as a 5-10 mg/kg IV infusion over 8-10 minutes to avert the nausea/vomiting and hypotension associated with rapid (bolus) administration.	2206, 2223
11	B	Lidocaine is a ventricular antidysrhythmic that is administered as a 1-1.5 mg/kg IV *bolus* in VF. Prophylactic lidocaine is not recommended in uncomplicated MI or ischemia *without* ventricular ectopy.	Updated since JAMA publication.
12	D	Defibrillation should be performed prior to an intubation attempt for the patient in VF.	2211, 2215
13	C	Isoproterenol is a pure β-adrenergic stimulating agent. Effects of administration include increased heart rate (chronotropy), increased force of contraction (inotropy) and vasodilation.	2207
14	B	Assess ABCs, perform CPR until a defibrillator is available, then defibrillate with 200J.	2216
15	C	Verapamil is a calcium channel blocker used in the treatment of stable patients with PSVT and in atrial fibrillation and flutter to control the ventricular response. Verapamil slows conduction and increases refractoriness in the AV node.	2207
16	D	Adenosine is useful in the management of narrow-QRS PSVT and is a second-line agent in the management of wide-complex tachycardia of uncertain origin.	2207

17	D	Dopamine's effects are dose-related: • 1-2 μg/kg/min $\rightarrow$ renal and mesenteric vasodilation • 2-10 μg/kg/min $\rightarrow$ β-adrenergic receptor stimulating effects (increased force of contraction, increased heart rate) $\rightarrow$ increased cardiac output • > 10 μg/kg/min $\rightarrow$ α-adrenergic receptor stimulating effects $\rightarrow$ vasoconstriction	2209
18	A	Emergent pacing is not indicated in cases of VF.	2214
19	B	This patient is unstable (chest pain, hypotension, altered level of consciousness and difficulty breathing). Administer oxygen, establish an IV, administer sedation, and then deliver synchronized countershock at 50 joules. Reassess the patient, rhythm and pulse. "If the patient displays serious signs and symptoms, prepare for immediate cardioversion".	2224
20	B	Heredity is a non-modifiable risk factor (as are age, gender and race).	2175
21	C	Aspirin is strongly recommended (Class I) for routine use in all MI patients as it has been shown to significantly improve mortality and decrease the incidence of reinfarction when used within 24 hours of onset of chest pain.	2231
22	D	Approximately 25 pounds of pressure should be applied when using conventional defibrillator paddles. This helps to maximize the surface area contact of the paddle against the patient's chest wall and helps to force exhalation - decreasing the distance within the chest.	2212
23	D	Guidelines for the management of pulseless electrical activity do not include the use of lidocaine.	2219
24	D	Sudden death related to coronary artery disease is the most prominent medical emergency in the U.S. today.	2174

25	A	Dopamine stimulates alpha, beta and dopaminergic receptors.	2209
26	C	The rhythm is second degree AV block, Type I (Mobitz I, Wenckebach). There are more P's than QRS's, the ventricular rhythm is irregular and the PR intervals lengthen until a P wave appears without a QRS.	N/A
27	D	Simultaneous, bilateral carotid pressure should NEVER be applied when performing carotid massage.	2224
28	B	Endpoints of procainamide administration include: • **hypotension** develops • the dysrhythmia is suppressed • a maximum of 17 mg/kg has been administered • the QRS complex widens more than 50% of its original width	2226
29	C	The unstable patient in monomorphic VT with a pulse should receive countershock at 100-200-300-360J.	2212, 2224
30	C	If a pacemaker is unavailable, an infusion of dopamine at 5-20 μg/kg/min should be initiated.	2221
31	B	The oropharyngeal airway should only be used in unconscious patients as it may stimulate vomiting or laryngospasm in the conscious patient. If improperly inserted, the OPA may press the epiglottis against the entrance of the larynx or may compress the tongue into the posterior pharynx, resulting in airway obstruction. When possible, the OPA should be inserted in unconscious patients who are not intubated.	2201
32	D	Advantages of the central venous route over the peripheral route include more rapid arrival of medications at their sites of action and successful placement, even when perfusion is poor.	2205

33	B	1 liter/min = 25% 4 liters/min = 37% 2 liters/min = 29% 5 liters/min = 41% 3 liters/min = 33% 6 liters/min = 45%	N/A
34	D	Lidocaine 1-1.5 mg/kg IV bolus is the first drug administered in wide complex tachycardia of uncertain origin.	2223, 2225
35	C	This patient is unstable (chest pain, hypotension, decreased level of consciousness). Administer a synchronized countershock at 50J. Reassess the patient, pulse and rhythm.	2224
36	A	Quinidine, disopyramide (Norpace), procainamide (Pronestyl) and other drugs that prolong repolarization are contraindicated because they can exacerbate torsades. Magnesium sulfate is the drug of choice. Isoproterenol is considered a Class IIa (possibly helpful) intervention in the management of this dysrhythmia. "Defibrillation should be used for any sustained episode of torsades."	2226
37	C	Norepinephrine increases myocardial oxygen demand and should be used with caution in patients with ischemic heart disease.	2209
38	D	Furosemide and sublingual nitroglycerin may be used in the management of acute pulmonary edema without hypotension.	2229
39	C	Dobutamine is a synthetic catecholamine useful in the treatment of heart failure. It stimulates β-adrenergic receptors and frequently induces reflex peripheral vasodilation. β-stimulation results in increased myocardial contractility.	2209
40	B	Continue ventilation with a bag-valve device and 100% oxygen, administer a lidocaine bolus and reassess the patient.	2206
41	C	Pop-off valves are not recommended since higher than usual airway pressures are often needed to ventilate patients in cardiac arrest. Pop-off valves may prevent the creation of airway pressures sufficient to overcome the increase in airway resistance.	2200

42	B	Lidocaine is indicated in the management of ventricular tachycardia, ventricular fibrillation, and wide complex tachycardia of uncertain origin. Lidocaine may be lethal if administered for an idioventricular (ventricular escape) rhythm.	2222
43	C	Verapamil is indicated in the management of stable but symptomatic patient with a NARROW-QRS complex supraventricular tachydysrhythmia or wide-complex tachycardia KNOWN WITH CERTAINTY to be supraventricular in origin. Verapamil should be administered over 3-4 minutes when treating the elderly or when the BP is within the lower range of normal. Verapamil should be used cautiously in patients who receive long-term β-blocker therapy.	2225
44	A	Lidocaine, epinephrine and atropine may be administered via the ET tube.	2205
45	B	Normal saline or lactated Ringer's solution are the preferred intravenous solutions for administration to the suspected stroke patient (unless hypoglycemia is STRONGLY suspected) because 5% dextrose in water is hypotonic and may increase cerebral edema.	2243
46	D	Class III = not indicated, may be harmful	2174
47	B	Atropine may be useful in symptomatic sinus bradycardia, AV block at the nodal level, pulseless electrical activity and asystole.	2207
48	A	True. Countershock and cardioversion are general terms. Unsynchronized countershock (or unsynchronized cardioversion) are synonymous with defibrillation and refers to the RANDOM delivery of energy during the cardiac cycle. Synchronized countershock (or synchronized cardioversion) refers to the PROGRAMMED delivery of energy within milliseconds of the R wave in the cardiac cycle.	2226

| 49 | C | The absolute refractory period begins with the onset of the QRS complex and terminates at approximately the apex of the T wave. During this period, the cell cannot propagate or conduct an impulse. | N/A |
| 50 | B | The recommendations for bicarbonate vary, depending on the clinical situation. When used, 1 mEq/kg should be administered as the initial dose, then half this dose every 10 minutes thereafter. | 2211 |

1 Adult Basic Life Support

ADULT ONE-RESCUER CPR

1.	Determine Responsiveness and Activate the EMS System (911)	Tap or gently shake the victim and shout, "Are you OK?" Activate the EMS system • 80-90% of adults are found to be in VF in cases of sudden non-traumatic cardiac arrest • Early activation of the EMS system, early bystander CPR and early defibrillation are keys to survival If trauma to the head and neck is visible or suspected, the victim should be moved only if absolutely necessary.
2.	Airway	• Head tilt-chin lift maneuver (preferred) • Jaw thrust maneuver (alternative for EMTs and other health care providers)
3.	Breathing (Assess 3-5 seconds)	Look For rise and fall of the chest Listen For air escaping during exhalation Feel For the flow of air • If the victim is breathing, place in the recovery position. • If the victim is not breathing, deliver two slow breaths, each lasting $1^{1}/_{2}$-2 seconds.

4. Circulation (Assess 5-10 seconds)	Check for a carotid pulse If a carotid pulse is PRESENT but the victim is not breathing, deliver one breath every 5-6 seconds (10-12/minute). If a carotid pulse is ABSENT, begin chest compressions. <ul><li>Position hands on the lower half of the sternum</li><li>Depress the sternum approximately 1$^{1}/_{2}$-2 inches (average adult)</li><li>Perform 15 external chest compressions for every 2 ventilations at a rate of 80-100 per minute ("one and, two and, three and, four and, . . .)</li><li>Open the airway and deliver two slow rescue breaths (each lasting 1.5-2 seconds)</li><li>Relocate proper hand position and begin 15 more compressions at a rate of 80-100 per minute</li><li>Perform four complete cycles of 15 compressions and 2 ventilations</li></ul>
5. Reassessment	After four cycles of compressions and ventilations (15:2 ratio), reassess the patient, checking the carotid pulse for 3-5 seconds. If a pulse is not felt, resume CPR and reassess pulse and breathing every few minutes. If a pulse IS present, check for breathing. <ul><li>If breathing IS present, continue monitoring the victim's pulse and breathing.</li><li>If breathing IS NOT present, continue rescue breathing at a rate of 10-12 breaths per minute and monitor the pulse.</li></ul>
6. Recovery position	If the victim resumes breathing and regains a pulse (and trauma is not apparent or suspected), roll the victim onto his/her side so that the head, shoulders and torso move simultaneously without twisting.

ADULT TWO-RESCUER CPR

1. Entrance of Second Rescuer to Replace the First Rescuer	• Second rescuer to activate the EMS system (if not previously done) • On arrival of the second rescuer, reassess breathing and pulse before CPR is resumed • Second rescuer should perform one-rescuer CPR when the first rescuer becomes fatigued
2. CPR Performed by Two Rescuers	• When possible, mouth-to-mask should be used • Rescuer at the victim's head maintains an open airway, monitors the carotid pulse for adequacy of chest compressions and provides rescue breathing • Compression rate is 80-100 per minute • Compression/ventilation ratio is 5:1 with a pause for ventilation (inspiration) of 1.5 to 2 seconds

FOREIGN BODY AIRWAY MANAGEMENT

Causes

Usually occurs during eating

In adults, meat is the most common cause of obstruction

Common factors associated with choking on food include:

- Large, poorly chewed pieces of food
- Elevated blood alcohol levels
- Dentures

PARTIAL AIRWAY OBSTRUCTION

Good Air
Exchange

Victim remains conscious

Can cough forcefully

Wheezing may be present between coughs

Management
- Encourage victim to continue spontaneous coughing and breathing efforts
- Do not interfere with victim's own attempts to expel the foreign body
- Stay with the victim
- If obstruction persists, activate the EMS system

Poor Air
Exchange

Weak, ineffective cough

High-pitched noise while inhaling

Increased respiratory difficulty

Possible cyanosis

Management
Treat as if a complete airway obstruction exists

COMPLETE AIRWAY OBSTRUCTION

Signs and
Symptoms

Unable to speak, breathe or cough

May clutch the neck with the thumb and fingers (universal distress signal)

Victim Standing or Sitting - Management	• Ask, "Are you choking?"
	• Assure victim you are going to assist him/her.
	• Stand behind victim
	    • Wrap your arms around the victim's waist.
	    • Make a fist with one hand (thumbside placed against the victim's abdomen in the midline slightly above the navel and well below the tip of the xiphoid).
	    • Grasp the fist with your other hand and deliver quick, upward thrusts.
	    • Continue until the object is expelled or the victim becomes unconscious.

If the victim is markedly obese or in cases of advanced pregnancy:

- Stand behind the victim and deliver chest thrusts
  - Bend your arms directly under the victim's armpits and encircle the victim's chest
  - Place the thumbside of one fist on the middle of the victim's sternum
  - Grab the fist with the other hand and perform chest thrusts
  - Continue until the foreign body is expelled or the victim becomes unconscious

Victim Lying- Management	• Kneel astride victim's thighs • Place heel of one hand against the victim's abdomen in the midline and well below the tip of the xiphoid • Place the second hand directly over the first • Deliver up to 5 quick, upward thrusts • Open airway and attempt to ventilate • Repeat sequence until effective

If the victim is markedly obese or in cases of advanced pregnancy:

- Place victim supine and kneel close to the victim's side
- Hand position is the same as that for chest compressions

Unconscious Adult	1. Open the airway and attempt to ventilate 2. If unsuccessful, reposition the airway and reattempt to ventilate 3. If unsuccessful, perform up to 5 abdominal thrusts 4. Perform a tongue-jaw lift and visualize the airway. Perform finger to remove the object 5. Repeat sequence until effective

ACLS In Perspective 2

Upon completion of this chapter, you will be able to:

1. Define "sudden death".
2. Describe the incidence of sudden death.
3. Identify the primary mechanisms of cardiac arrest.
4. Identify the current classification of therapeutic interventions.
5. Identify and describe the four components of the chain of survival.
6. List three non-modifiable risk factors for atherosclerosis.
7. List five modifiable risk factors for atherosclerosis.
8. Define "cardiopulmonary-cerebral resuscitation".
9. Identify the components of emergency cardiac care.
10. List five life-threatening events that may not initially involve the heart.
11. Identify the purpose of basic life support.
12. Identify the components of advanced cardiac life support.

SUDDEN DEATH

Definition

Unexpected death of cardiac etiology occurring either immediately or within one hour of onset of symptoms

The Problem

- Sudden death related to coronary artery disease is the most prominent medical emergency in the U.S. today
- Approximately 2/3 of sudden deaths due to coronary disease take place outside the hospital
- Usually occurs within 2 hours after onset of symptoms

Signs/Symptoms

- Usually occur in patients with a history of ischemic heart disease
- Cardiac arrest may be first evidence of disease in up to 20% of patients
- Majority of patients who suffer sudden death have no premonitory symptoms immediately prior to collapse

Out-of-Hospital Cardiac Arrest

Primary mechanisms of cardiac arrest:

- VF most common
- VT
- Bradycardia, asystole, pulseless electrical activity
- Supraventricular tachydysrhythmias may be another mechanism of cardiac arrest[1]

Statistics

1. Decline in mortality since 1972

   From 1979-1989, the death rate from coronary heart disease decreased 30% and the death rate from stroke decreased 31.5%

2. Cardiovascular disease accounts for nearly 1 million deaths annually in the U.S. (nearly 50% of deaths from all causes)

3. Approximately 500,000 deaths due to coronary disease, a majority of which are sudden deaths

4. More than 160,000 of these deaths occur before the age of 65 years

5. More than 1/2 of all deaths from cardiovascular disease occur in women

6. 45% of all heart attacks occur in people less than 65 years of age

7. 1989 statistics estimate 6.2 million Americans have significant coronary heart disease

Classification of Therapeutic Interventions

Where possible, the American Heart Associations recommendations are based on the strength of supporting scientific evidence[2] and classified as follows:

Class I -   Definitely helpful
Class IIa - Probably helpful
Class IIb - Possibly helpful
Class III - Not indicated, may be harmful

CHAIN OF SURVIVAL

Four Components:

• Early Access
• Early CPR
• Early Defibrillation
• Early ACLS

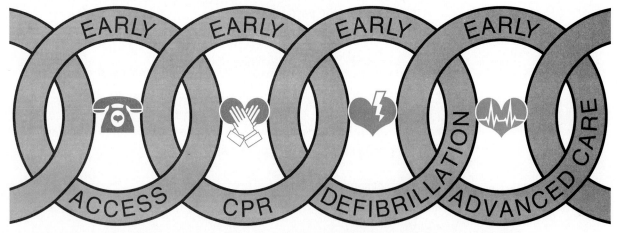

Figure 2-1   The Chain of Survival. (Reproduced with permission of *JAMA*, October 28, 1992 - Vol. 268, No. 16)

EARLY ACCESS

Public Education

- Recognition of the early warning signs of a heart attack and the need for prompt attention
- Early recognition of patient collapse
- How to gain rapid access to the EMS system (usually by telephone) via EMS dispatchers

AHA Recommendations:

- Obtaining a 911 system for all communities (preferably enhanced 911) is a Class I recommendation
  - Enhanced 911 automatically provides dispatchers with the caller's address and telephone number
- Rapid recognition by EMS dispatchers of a potential cardiac arrest
- Rapid dispatch instructions to EMS responders
- Rapid arrival of EMS responders at the appropriate incident site
- EMS responder arrival at the site with all necessary equipment
- Identification of an arrest

EARLY CPR

- In most situations, bystander CPR greatly affects survival (possible exception when call-to-defibrillation period extremely short)
- Bystander CPR best treatment patient can receive until arrival of defibrillator and ACLS
- CPR training teaches citizens how to contact the EMS system, decreasing the time to defibrillation
- Bystander CPR rarely causes significant injury to victims
- In an adult victim arrest, the bystander should determine unresponsiveness, call 911 and then initiate CPR
- In pediatric arrest, the EMS system should be activated after 1 minute of rescue efforts

Methods of increasing the availability of early CPR:

- CPR training programs for targeted groups (teaching families of patients at high risk)
- Dispatcher-assisted CPR
- Community-wide CPR training programs

EARLY
DEFIBRILLATION

Link most likely to improve survival

AHA Recommendations:

1. Automated External Defibrillators (AEDs) should be widely available for appropriately trained people.
2. All fire-fighting units that perform CPR and first aid should be equipped with, and trained to operate, AEDs.
3. AEDs should be placed in gathering places of more than 10,000 people.
4. Legislation should be enacted to allow all EMS personnel to perform early defibrillation.

EARLY ACLS

- EMS systems should provide a minimum of 2 ACLS trained rescuers to respond to an emergency
    - Increased survival rates associated with EMS systems that have a minimum of 2 ACLS providers AND a minimum of 2 BLS providers at the scene
    - Every EMS system should strive for a 2 ACLS and 2 BLS EMS provider level of response
- Besides defibrillation, intubation and IV administration of medications may significantly improve cardiac arrest outcome

COMMUNITY EDUCATION

1. Greatest risk of death from heart attack occurs within the first 2 hours after onset of symptoms
2. Success of thrombolytic agents in decreasing mortality and morbidity of acute MI has increased the urgency for early care

Public education must include:

1. Recognition of usual signs of a heart attack and need for prompt attention
2. How to rapidly access the EMS system (911)
3. Plan of action for use in an emergency, based on community resources and the EMS system

RISK FACTOR MODIFICATION

Non-modifiable
Risk Factors

Heredity
Male Gender
Race
Age

Modifiable
Risk Factors

1. Cigarette smoking
   - Most important single cause of preventable death in the U.S.
2. Hypertension
   - Systolic blood pressure of 160 mm Hg or more or diastolic BP of 95 mm Hg or more associated with increased risk of coronary artery disease
   - A major risk factor for coronary heart disease
   - The major risk factor for left ventricular hypertrophy (which is thought to be an independent cause of dysrhythmia and sudden death)
   - Control of hypertension dramatically reduces incidence of stroke
3. Elevated cholesterol levels
   - Increased total cholesterol → increased risk of coronary artery disease
4. Elevated triglyceride levels
   - Increased serum triglyceride associated with increased risk of coronary artery disease, especially in women
5. Lack of exercise
   - Regular physical activity decreases risk of coronary artery disease
6. Obesity
   - Associated with numerous risk factors including hypertension, diabetes and hypercholesterolemia
7. Stress
   - Stress reduction techniques decrease blood pressure
8. Diabetes

Independent Risk
Factors

A 1992 study attempted "to determine if the presence of a disrupted marriage or living alone would be a prognostic risk factor for a subsequent major cardiac event following an initial myocardial infarction."[3]

This study demonstrated that living alone was associated with a recurrent cardiac event rate of 15.8% at six months. This was compared to patients living with others, who had a recurrent rate of 8.8%. The study also demonstrated that "a disrupted marriage was not an independent risk factor."

RESPONSIBILITY TO THE FUTURE

Goal of the CPR-Emergency Cardiac Care Program

To increase the number of persons reached and adequately trained, thereby increasing the number of lives saved by prevention, risk factor modification and emergency intervention, and to do so at the most efficient cost

Survival Related to Response Times

- BLS is often successful if defibrillation or other modes of definitive care can be carried out within 8-10 minutes
- If CPR or definitive care is delayed, the cerebral cortex is irreversibly damaged, resulting in severe neurological deficit or death

EMERGENCY CARDIAC CARE

Components of Emergency Cardiac Care

1. "Recognizing early warning signs of heart attack, efforts to prevent complications, reassurance of the victim, and prompt availability of monitoring equipment
2. Providing immediate BLS at the scene when needed
3. Providing ACLS at the scene as quickly as possible to defibrillate, if necessary, and stabilize the victim before transportation
4. Transferring the stabilized victim to an appropriate hospital where definitive cardiac care can be provided"[4]

Special Resuscitation Situations

Life-threatening events that may not initially involve the heart:
- Obstructed airway
- Stroke
- Near-drowning
- Electrocution
- Trauma
- Hypothermia
- Pediatric resuscitation
- Neonatal resuscitation

Phases of Emergency Cardiac Care

1. Basic Life Support (BLS)
2. Advanced Cardiac Life Support (ACLS)

Basic Life Support
(BLS)

1. Attempts to prevent arrested or inadequate circulation or respiration through prompt recognition and intervention, early entry into the EMS system, or both.

2. Attempts to provide respiratory and circulatory support to the arrested victim through CPR

3. Should be initiated by any person present when cardiac or respiratory arrest occurs

4. Most important link in the CPR-Emergency Cardiac Care system in the community is the layperson

   - Dependent upon layperson's understanding of importance of early activation of EMS system and on willingness and ability to promptly initiate effective CPR

Advanced Cardiac
Life Support
(ACLS)

1. Includes BLS *plus*:
   - adjunctive equipment in supporting ventilation
   - establishment of IV access
   - administration of drugs
   - cardiac monitoring
   - defibrillation or other control of dysrhythmias
   - care after resuscitation
   - establishment of communication necessary to ensure continued care

2. Physician must supervise and direct ACLS efforts via one of the following:
   - in person at the scene
   - by direct communication
   - by a previously defined alternate mechanism such as standing orders (protocols)

General Concepts
of Resuscitation
Education

1. Emergency Cardiac Care courses are strictly educational

2. The term "certification" has been removed from provider cards and replaced with "course completion"

3. A course completion document may be issued to a participant who has:
   - attended the required course
   - achieved a successful evaluation on the core content
   - remedied any deficiencies when the course was given

4. The term "standards" has been replaced with "guidelines" and "recommendations"

REFERENCES

1. Wang Y, Scheinman MM, Chien WW, Cohen TJ, Lesh MD, Griffin JC: Patients with supraventricular tachycardia presenting with aborted sudden death: incidence, mechanism, and long-term followup, *J Am Coll Cardiol* 18:1711-1719, 1991.

2. Emergency Cardiac Care Committee and Subcommittees, American Heart Association. Guidelines for cardiopulmonary resuscitation and emergency cardiac care. *JAMA* 268:2174, 1992.

3. Case RB, Moss AJ, Case N, McDermott M, Eberly S: Living alone after myocardial infarction: Impact on prognosis. *JAMA* 267:515-519, 1992.

4. Emergency Cardiac Care Committee and Subcommittees, American Heart Association. Guidelines for cardiopulmonary resuscitation and emergency cardiac care. *JAMA* 268:2177, 1992.

Myocardial Infarction

3

Upon completion of this chapter, you will be able to:

1. Define "myocardial infarction."
2. Identify the ECG changes that may be associated with acute myocardial infarction.
3. Describe the terms "transmural" and "subendocardial" MI.
4. Describe the classic signs and symptoms that are associated with acute myocardial infarction.
5. Describe the initial management of acute myocardial infarction.
6. Explain why pain relief is a high priority in the management of acute myocardial infarction.
7. Explain the benefits of thrombolytic therapy.
8. Describe the management of each of the following:
   - Premature ventricular complexes
   - Symptomatic bradycardia
   - Supraventricular tachycardia (PSVT)
   - Ventricular tachycardia
   - Ventricular fibrillation
   - Wide-complex tachycardia of uncertain origin
   - Pulseless electrical activity
   - Asystole
   - Acute MI with hypotension
   - Acute MI with pulmonary edema
   - Acute MI with hypertension

ACUTE MYOCARDIAL INFARCTION

Definitions

Myocardial infarction

- Necrosis of some mass of heart muscle due to inadequate blood supply

ECG Changes in Acute Myocardial Infarction

- Zone of ischemia → inverted T wave due to altered repolarization
- Zone of injury → elevated ST segment due to severe ischemia
- Zone of infarction → abnormal Q wave due to lack of depolarization of necrotic tissue

Transmural MI

- Entire thickness of the myocardium is destroyed
- Often called Q-wave (producing) infarction as it usually produces, or is associated with changes in, the Q wave on the ECG
- ST segments are often elevated and T waves may be deeply inverted
- Generally accepted criteria for diagnostic Q waves:
  - More than 0.04 sec in duration
  - More than 1/4 of the height of the R wave in the same lead

Subendocardial MI

- Subendocardial layer involved, does not extend through to the epicardial wall
- Often called non-Q-wave (producing) infarction
- Less often associated with thrombosis
- Early stages of subendocardial MI often characterized by depressed or elevated ST segments
- T waves may be inverted

Localization of MI

1. Anterior infarction
   - Occlusion of the proximal left anterior descending coronary artery
2. Anterolateral infarction
   - Occlusion of the left circumflex, marginal branch of the left circumflex or diagonal branch of the left anterior descending artery
3. Diaphragmatic or inferior infarction
   - Occlusion of the right coronary artery
4. True posterior infarction
   - Occlusion of the left distal circumflex, left posterior descending or distal right coronary arteries

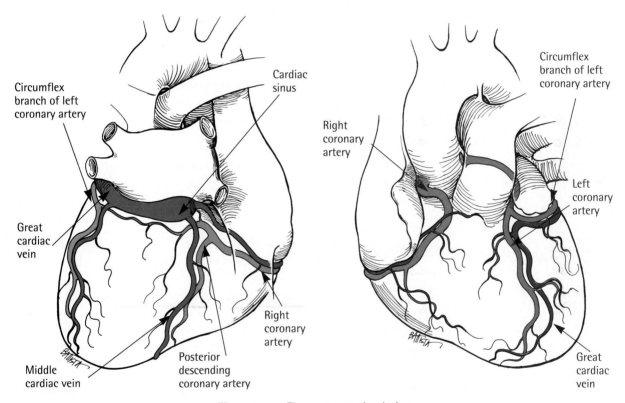

Figure 3-1   The coronary circulation.

Precipitating Events

- Rest, sleep or usual activities
- Morning hours (6:00 a.m. to noon)

Sign/Symptom Recognition

- Pain often described as crushing, squeezing, pressing, or heavy
- Pain may radiate to one (more often the left) or both shoulders and arms, neck, jaw or back
- In a high-risk person, unusual or prolonged "indigestion" should raise suspicion of MI
- Chest pain is frequently associated with MI, however, in a study of the elderly population, roughly 2/3 did not experience chest pain[1]

EARLY MANAGEMENT – GENERAL PRINCIPLES

Diagnosis and Early
Treatment

1. Based on the patient's history and presenting signs and symptoms
2. Initial ECG is not conclusive
   - The initial ECG is diagnostic of acute injury in only 24-60% of patients with a final diagnosis of acute myocardial infarction[2]

Oxygen Therapy

1. Hypoxemia leads to anaerobic metabolism and metabolic acidosis, reducing the effectiveness of pharmacologic and electrical therapy
2. Supplemental O_2 decreases the extent of ST-segment changes in patients experiencing an acute MI
3. Lower O_2 flow rates (1-2 liters/min) may be necessary for COPD patients, however, "Oxygen should not be withheld for fear of suppressing respiration if hypoxemia is suspected or if significant respiratory distress is present. The rescuer should be prepared to provide assisted ventilation if necessary."[3]

ECG Monitoring

1. Should be initiated immediately
2. High incidence of VF and other serious dysrhythmias during the early hours of infarction
   - The most common cause of death within the first hours of an MI is cardiac dysrhythmias
3. ST-segment elevation of 0.1 mV or more in two or more adjacent leads is considered indicative of myocardial injury due to acute ischemia[4]

IV Access

1. Large-bore IV line of normal saline or Lactated Ringer's solution
2. Antecubital vein
   - If pulseless and no IV line is in place at the time of arrest, the antecubital or external jugular veins are sites of first choice

Pain Relief   Relief of pain is a high priority

1. Benefits

   - Decreases anxiety and pain
   - May decrease BP and heart rate
   - Decreases myocardial oxygen demand
   - Decreases risk of dysrhythmias

2. Therapy

   - Sublingual nitroglycerin (if normotensive or hypertensive) 1 tablet (0.3 mg or 0.4 mg), repeated as needed every 5 minutes (maximum of 3 tablets)
   - IV nitroglycerin for severe acute ischemic chest pain and blood pressure > 100 mm Hg
     - Increases venous capacitance (decreases preload)
     - Arteriole vasodilation (decreases afterload)
     - Coronary artery vasodilation
   - Morphine (if nitro unsuccessful or pain is severe) in small IV doses (1-3 mg), repeated every 5 min, titrated to pain relief

3. Complications

   - Hypotension
   - Dysrhythmias due to myocardial hypoperfusion or reperfusion

Thrombolytic Therapy

1. High incidence of total coronary occlusion due to coronary thrombosis early in MI

2. Early administration may decrease morbidity and mortality in patients with acute transmural MI

3. Should be considered for all patients with symptoms and ECG findings of acute MI (if no reason for exclusion)

4. Should be administered as soon as possible after onset of symptoms by the first physician competent in making the diagnosis of acute MI

5. All patients receiving thrombolytics should receive 150-325 mg of aspirin (decreases mortality and reinfarction)

6. Early IV β-blockade may decrease reinfarction and incidence of intracranial bleeding in patients receiving thrombolytics

   - IV β-blockers should NOT be administered to patients with hypotension, AV block, congestive heart failure, bradycardia or history of bronchospastic disease

7. No significant difference in safety and efficacy between t-PA, urokinase, APSAC and streptokinase

Infarct Limitation

1. Diltiazem (calcium channel blocker)
   - May decrease incidence of early recurrent reinfarction in non-Q-wave MI
   - Not helpful in Q-wave MI and significant left ventricular dysfunction

2. IV Nitroglycerin
   - Increases collateral blood flow to ischemic areas with a secondary potential benefit on infarct size
   - Use in patients with persistent chest pain, without hypovolemia and without right ventricular infarction

3. β-Blockers
   - In hemodynamically STABLE patients with acute MI who did not receive thrombolytic agents, either atenolol (5 mg IV over 5 min) or metoprolol (5-10 mg slow IV push at 5 min intervals to a total of 15 mg) may be administered
   - IV β-blockers should NOT be administered to patients with hypotension, AV block, congestive heart failure, bradycardia or history of bronchospastic disease

4. Aspirin
   - Has been shown to significantly improve mortality and decrease the incidence of reinfarction when used within 24 hours of onset of chest pain[5]
   - Routine use in all MI patients strongly recommended (Class I)

Prophylactic
Antidysrhythmic
Therapy

1. Routine use of prophylactic antidysrhythmic agents no longer recommended
   - In 1986, the AHA recommended lidocaine be administered as early as possible following the onset of symptoms, even in the absence of PVCs, and continued for at least 24 hours
   - Several studies questioned this recommendation. Lidocaine studies "not only failed to demonstrate improved prognosis, but in some cases, have cited a small but important occurrence rate of asystole and other adverse reactions after prophylactic lidocaine administration."[6]
2. Prophylactic antidysrhythmic use should be avoided in patients older than 70 years due to increased incidence of lidocaine toxicity
3. Patients seen more than six hours after onset of chest pain are less likely to develop VF, therefore routine lidocaine therapy not advisable in these patients

DYSRHYTHMIA COMPLICATIONS - PVCS

The Problem

1. PVCs common with acute MI
2. Prophylactic lidocaine administration no longer recommended

Therapy

- Lidocaine should be avoided as a routine treatment for PVCs
- In the patient with an acute MI/ischemia, treatment should be directed at rapid identification and correction of electrolyte abnormalities
  - Hypokalemia (serum K+ < 3.5 mEq/L)
  - Hypomagnesemia (serum Mg++ level < 1.4 mEq/L)
- Consider the use of beta-blockers (if not contraindicated) and magnesium
- If unsuccessful, or if significant ventricular ectopy present, lidocaine may be used
  - Initial dose 1-1.5 mg/kg IV bolus
  - May repeat as needed with 0.5-0.75 mg/kg every 5-10 minutes to a maximum total dose of 3 mg/kg

DYSRHYTHMIA COMPLICATIONS – BRADYCARDIAS

The Problem

1. Common during the first hours of symptoms
2. May include:
   - Sinus bradycardia
   - Junctional rhythm
   - AV block (at the level of the AV node)
   - Second or third-degree AV block at the ventricular level
   - New bundle branch block

When to Treat

1. If no symptoms, hypotension or PVCs, no treatment
2. Treatment is indicated if ventricular rate is less than 60 beats/min and:
   - symptoms (chest pain, dyspnea)
   - hypotension or
   - ventricular ectopy present

Therapy

1. Narrow-QRS bradycardia → atropine
   - Atropine is a Class I intervention in sinus bradycardia (definitely helpful)
   - Atropine is a Class IIa (probably helpful) intervention in AV block at the nodal level
2. Wide-QRS AV block bradycardia or new bundle branch block → pacing

DYSRHYTHMIA COMPLICATIONS – AV BLOCKS

First Degree AV Block

1. No treatment unless symptomatic bradycardia
2. Monitor for progression

Second Degree AV Block, Type I (Wenckebach, Mobitz I)

1. Block usually occurs at the level of the AV node
   - Resulting QRS is usually narrow (<.10 sec) since the level of the block is above the branching portion of the bundle of His
2. May occur because of:
   - Increased parasympathetic tone
   - Inferior wall MI
   - Effects of drugs such as digitalis, propranolol, verapamil
3. No treatment unless symptomatic
4. If symptomatic:
   a. Atropine 0.5-1.0 mg every 3-5 min
      - maximum dose 0.03-0.04 mg/kg (2-3 mg in 70 kg patient)
   b. Transcutaneous pacing
   c. Dopamine infusion 5-20 μg/kg/min
   d. Epinephrine infusion 2-10 μg/min
   e. Isoproterenol infusion (low dose)

Second Degree AV Block, Type II (Mobitz II)

1. Usually occurs at the level of the bundle branches
   - Resulting QRS is usually wide (>.10 sec) since the level of the block often involves the bundle of His
2. Usually associated with anteroseptal MI
3. May rapidly progress to third degree AV block without warning
4. Preparations for a transvenous pacer should be made as soon as this rhythm is identified
5. Transcutaneous pacing may be used until transvenous pacing can be accomplished
6. Atropine use *may* increase sinus node activity; however, the impulses bombarding an ischemic AV junction may result in increased AV block, further decreasing heart rate and blood pressure.

Third Degree
(Complete) AV
Block

May occur at the level of the AV node OR the bundle of His

1. If the block is at the level of the AV node → usually junctional escape pacer → narrow QRS (inferior MI)

   • If symptomatic: atropine, transcutaneous pacing, dopamine, epi-nephrine (possible isoproterenol)

2. If the block is at the level of the bundle of His → ventricular escape pacer → wide QRS (anterior MI)

   • If symptomatic: transcutaneous pacing until transvenous pacing can be accomplished

DYSRHYTHMIA COMPLICATIONS – SUPRAVENTRICULAR TACHYCARDIAS

The Problem

Tachycardia may increase the area of infarction or exacerbate ischemia

Sinus Tachycardia

Identify and correct cause:

• Pain = analgesia

• Hypovolemia = volume replacement

• Extensive myocardial damage = hemodynamic monitoring and drug therapy

ATRIAL FLUTTER AND ATRIAL FIBRILLATION
WITH A RAPID VENTRICULAR RESPONSE

Stable patient

Assess ABCs
↓
Administer oxygen
↓
Establish IV access
↓
For rate control
β-blockers (esmolol, metoprolol, propranolol)
Calcium channel blockers (diltiazem, verapamil)
Digitalis (of questionable value in the emergent treatment
of atrial fibrillation and atrial flutter)

For pharmacologic conversion
Procainamide
Quinidine

Caution: IV propranolol should not be administered after IV verapamil. May result
in profound bradycardia and possible asystole when given < 30 min
apart.

**Unstable patient –
Atrial Flutter**

ABCs, O_2, IV
↓
Consider medications
↓
If the patient displays serious signs and symptoms,
prepare for immediate countershock
↓
Administer sedation whenever possible
↓
Synchronized countershock with 50J, 100J, 200J, 300J, 360J

**Unstable patient –
Atrial Fibrillation**

ABCs, O_2, IV
↓
Consider medications
↓
If the patient displays serious signs and symptoms,
prepare for immediate countershock
↓
Administer sedation whenever possible
↓
Synchronized countershock with 100J, 200J, 300J, 360J

PAROXYSMAL SUPRAVENTRICULAR TACHYCARDIA (PSVT)

Stable patient

ABCs, O$_2$, IV
↓
Vagal maneuvers
↓
Adenosine 6 mg rapid IV bolus
Consider decreasing the dose in patients on dipyridamole (Persantine)
Consider increasing the dose in patients on theophylline
↓
If needed, after 1-2 minutes:
Adenosine 12 mg rapid IV bolus
↓
If needed, after 1-2 minutes:
Adenosine 12 mg rapid IV bolus
↓
Verapamil 2.5-5.0 mg slow IV bolus
↓
If needed, after 15-30 minutes:
Verapamil 5-10 mg slow IV bolus
↓
Consider Digoxin, β-blockers,
Diltiazem

Unstable patient

ABCs, O$_2$, IV
↓
Consider medications
↓
If the patient displays serious signs and symptoms,
prepare for immediate countershock
↓
Administer sedation whenever possible
↓
Synchronized countershock
50, 100J, 200J, 300J, 360J

DYSRHYTHMIA COMPLICATIONS –
WIDE-COMPLEX TACHYCARDIA OF UNCERTAIN ORIGIN

Stable Patient

ABCs, O$_2$, IV
↓
Lidocaine 1-1.5 mg/kg IV bolus
↓
In 5-10 minutes:
Lidocaine 0.5-0.75 mg/kg IV bolus every
5-10 min to maximum of 3 mg/kg
↓
Adenosine 6 mg rapid IV bolus
Consider decreasing the dose in patients on dipyridamole (Persantine)
Consider increasing the dose in patients on theophylline
↓
If needed, in 1-2 minutes:
Adenosine 12 mg rapid IV bolus
↓
If needed, in 1-2 minutes:
Adenosine 12 mg rapid IV bolus
↓
Procainamide 20-30 mg/min
Maximum dose 17 mg/kg
(approximately 1.2 grams in a 70 kg patient)
↓
Bretylium 5-10 mg/kg infusion
in 50 ml D5W over 8-10 min
Maximum 30 mg/kg over 24 hours
↓
Consider synchronized countershock

Caution: Administration of verapamil may be lethal unless the wide-complex
tachycardia is known WITH CERTAINTY to be supraventricular in origin[7]

Unstable Patient

ABCs, O$_2$, IV
↓
Consider medications
↓
If the patient displays serious signs and symptoms,
prepare for immediate countershock
↓
Administer sedation whenever possible
↓
Synchronized countershock with 100J, 200J, 300J, 360J

NOTE: If undue delay in synchronization, or if clinical conditions are critical,
UNSYNC (defibrillate) at same energy.

DYSRHYTHMIA COMPLICATIONS – VENTRICULAR TACHYCARDIA

Stable Patient	ABCs, O2, IV ↓ Lidocaine 1-1.5 mg/kg Repeat with 0.5-0.75 mg/kg every 5-10 minutes as needed to a maximum of 3 mg/kg ↓ Procainamide 20-30 mg/min to a maximum dose of 17 mg/kg ↓ Bretylium 5-10 mg/kg infusion over 8-10 minutes ↓ Synchronized countershock with 100J, 200J, 300J, 360J
Unstable Patient Signs/symptoms: • Dyspnea • Chest pain • Ischemia • Infarction • Hypotension • Pulmonary edema, congestive heart failure • Decreased level of consciousness	ABCs, O2, IV ↓ Consider medications ↓ If the patient displays serious signs and symptoms, prepare for immediate countershock ↓ Administer sedation whenever possible ↓ Synchronized countershock with 100J, 200J, 300J, 360J NOTE: If undue delay in synchronization, or if clinical conditions are critical, UNSYNC (defibrillate) at same energy
Pulseless VT	Treat as VF with unsynchronized countershock (defibrillation) 200J, 200-300J, 360J

POLYMORPHIC VENTRICULAR TACHYCARDIA	
Stable Patient	1. Treatment of choice is transcutaneous ("overdrive") pacing 2. Drug therapy • Magnesium sulfate 1-2 grams IV (2-4 ml of 50% solution) diluted in 10 ml administered over 1-2 minutes followed by same amount (mixed in 50-100 ml) infused over 1 hour (drug of choice) • Isoproterenol infusion at 2-10 μg/min
Unstable Patient (Sustained Rhythm)	ABCs, O$_2$, IV Administer sedation whenever possible Unsynchronized countershock with 200, 200-300, 360J

DYSRHYTHMIA COMPLICATIONS – VENTRICULAR FIBRILLATION

Management	

CPR until defibrillator available
Precordial thump (if witnessed)
Perform quick-look
↓
Defibrillate with 200J, 200-300J, 360J
Leave the paddles in place on the chest between shocks
(or use adhesive defibrillation pads for remote defibrillation)
Visually reconfirm rhythm between defibrillations
↓
Continue CPR
Intubate at once (confirm tube placement)
↓
IV access
Large-bore IV
Antecubital or external jugular vein if no IV in place at time of arrest
Normal saline or lactated Ringer's solution
↓
Epinephrine 1 mg IV every 3-5 minutes
(or, after initial dose, appropriate alternative*)
If IV access delayed, endotracheal (ET) dose is 2-2.5 mg
diluted in 10 ml of normal saline or distilled water
↓
Defibrillate with 360J within 30-60 sec
↓

IV Dosing Alternatives

Recommended: 1 mg
every 3-5 min

REFRACTORY VF
Lidocaine 1-1.5 mg/kg IV push
May repeat every 5-10 minutes to a maximum total dose of 3 mg/kg
↓
Defibrillate with 360J within 30-60 sec
↓

Intermediate: 2-5 mg IV
push, every 3-5 min

Bretylium 5 mg/kg
May repeat with 10 mg/kg every 5 minutes as needed to
a maximum dose of 30-35 mg/kg
↓
Defibrillate with 360J within 30-60 sec
↓

Escalating: 1 mg-3 mg-5
mg IV 3 min apart

Magnesium sulfate 1-2 grams IV (2-4 ml of 50% solution)
in 10 ml over 1-2 minutes
↓

High: 0.1 mg/kg IV push
every 3-5 min

Defibrillate with 360J within 30-60 sec
↓
Procainamide 30 mg/min (Maximum dose 17 mg/kg)
↓
Defibrillate with 360J within 30-60 sec
↓
Consider sodium bicarbonate 1 mEq/kg

Pattern should be drug-shock, drug-shock

Although it may take 1-2 minutes for drugs to reach the central circulation,
"successive shocks are more important than adjunctive drug therapy and delays
between shocks to deliver medications are detrimental"[8]

ASYSTOLE	
Management	CPR ↓ Intubate (Confirm tube placement) Assess breath sounds Observe chest rise ↓ Establish IV access Large bore IV Normal saline or lactated Ringer's Antecubital or external jugular ↓ Confirm rhythm in another lead Change lead-selector on the monitor If using paddles in quick-look mode, rotate paddles 90° ↓ Consider possible causes: **H(x4)AD** **H**ypoxia **H**ypokalemia **H**yperkalemia **H**ypothermia **A**cidosis (preexisting) **D**rug overdose ↓ Consider Immediate Transcutaneous Pacing ↓
IV Dosing Alternatives Recommended: 1 mg every 3-5 min Intermediate: 2-5 mg IV push, every 3-5 min Escalating: 1 mg-3 mg-5 mg IV 3 min apart High: 0.1 mg/kg IV push every 3-5 min	Epinephrine 1 mg IV every 3-5 minutes (or, after initial dose, appropriate alternative*) ET dose 2-2.5 mg diluted in 10 ml of normal saline or distilled water ↓ Atropine 1 mg IV every 3-5 minutes to maximum 0.04 mg/kg (approximately 3 mg in 70 kg patient) ET dose 2-2.5 mg diluted in 10 ml of normal saline or distilled water ↓ Consider sodium bicarbonate 1 mEq/kg ↓ Consider termination of efforts

Sodium Bicarbonate use:

Class I (definitely helpful) if known preexisting hyperkalemia
Class IIa (Probably helpful)
- If known preexisting bicarbonate-responsive acidosis
- If overdose with cyclic antidepressants
- To alkalinize the urine in drug overdoses

Class IIb (Possibly helpful)
- If intubated and long arrest interval
- Upon return of spontaneous circulation after long arrest interval

Class III (Not indicated, may be harmful)
- Hypoxic lactic acidosis

PULSELESS ELECTRICAL ACTIVITY

Includes:
Electromechanical dissociation (EMD)

Pseudo-EMD
- Electrical activity associated with myocardial contractions too weak to produce a palpated or auscultated blood pressure

Idioventricular (ventricular escape) rhythms
- Including postdefibrillation idioventricular rhythms

Bradyasystolic rhythms

IV Dosing Alternatives

Recommended: 1 mg every 3-5 min

Intermediate: 2-5 mg IV push, every 3-5 min

Escalating: 1 mg-3 mg-5 mg IV 3 min apart

High: 0.1 mg/kg IV push every 3-5 min

CPR
↓
Intubate (confirm tube placement)
Assess breath sounds
Observe chest rise
↓
Establish IV access
Large bore IV
Normal saline or lactated Ringer's
Antecubital or external jugular
500 ml fluid challenge
↓
Assess blood flow using Doppler
↓
Consider underlying causes
↓
MATCH(x4)ED
Myocardial Infarction (massive acute)
Acidosis (severe)
Tension pneumothorax
Peri**C**ardial tamponade
Hypoxia (severe)
Hypothermia
Hypovolemia
Hyperkalemia
Pulmonary **E**mbolism (massive)
Drug overdose
↓
Epinephrine 1 mg IV every 3-5 minutes
(or, after initial dose, appropriate alternative*)
ET dose 2-2.5 mg diluted in 10 ml of normal saline or distilled water
↓

If bradycardic, atropine 1 mg IV every 3-5 minutes
to maximum 3 mg
ET dose 2-2.5 mg diluted in 10 ml of normal saline or distilled water

↓
Consider sodium bicarbonate 1 mEq/kg

Sodium Bicarbonate use:

Class I (definitely helpful) if known preexisting hyperkalemia

Class IIa (Probably helpful)
- If known preexisting bicarbonate-responsive acidosis
- If overdose with cyclic antidepressants
- To alkalinize the urine in drug overdoses

Class IIb (Possibly helpful)
- If intubated and long arrest interval
- Upon return of spontaneous circulation after long arrest interval

Class III (Not indicated, may be harmful)
- Hypoxic lactic acidosis

HYPOTENSION AND SHOCK

Shock
- Inadequate cellular perfusion and inadequate oxygen delivery for existing metabolic demands common to all shock states.
- Signs and symptoms differ according to underlying cause and compensatory mechanisms.

Cardiovascular Triad
1. Conduction system
2. Vascular system (volume)
3. Myocardium (pump)

Hypotension

Hypotension occurs as a result of a problem with one of the components of the cardiovascular triad

Assessment

"For every patient with shock or hypotension, one should ask: is there a rate problem, a pump problem or a volume problem?"[9]

ACUTE MI WITH HYPOTENSION – RATE PROBLEMS

Rate Problem

Rate problem is NOT synonymous with "conducting problem"
- Adequate rate may be present although a conduction defect exists
- Assess patient for possible pump or volume problems if hypotensive but rate is normal

If a notable rate problem exists and unclear if significant pump or volume problem coexists, treat the heart rate first (ie, correct the heart rate of a hypotensive, bradycardic patient before administering a fluid challenge, vasopressor or inotrope).

If a rate problem coexists with suspected pump or volume problems, treat simultaneously

Therapy
1. ABCs, O_2, IV, cardiac monitor, pulse oximetry, assess vital signs, review history, physical examination, 12-lead ECG, portable chest roentgenogram
2. Rate too slow use bradycardia algorithm
3. Rate too fast use tachycardia algorithm

ACUTE MI WITH HYPOTENSION – VOLUME PROBLEMS

Causes

Absolute (actual fluid deficit)
- Hemorrhage
- Gastrointestinal loss (vomiting, diarrhea)
- Renal losses (polyuria)
- Insensible losses
  - Perspiration
  - Respiration
- Adrenal insufficiency (aldosterone)

Relative (vasodilation from any cause or redistribution of fluid to third spaces)
- Central nervous system injury
- Spinal injury
- Third-space loss
- Tension pneumothorax
- Adrenal insufficiency (cortisol)
- Sepsis
- Drugs that alter vascular tone
- Anaphylaxis

Therapy

ABCs, O_2, IV, cardiac monitor, pulse oximetry, assess vital signs, review history, physical examination, 12-lead ECG, portable chest roentgenogram

1. Generally, first priority = fluid replacement
   Administer fluids, blood transfusion to increase volume

2. Consider vasopressors, if indicated, to improve vascular tone

ACUTE MI WITH HYPOTENSION – PUMP PROBLEMS

Pump Problems

- May result in decreased cardiac output and may produce signs and symptoms of tissue hypoperfusion or pulmonary congestion.
- May be primary or secondary.

Signs and
Symptoms of
Hypoperfusion

Hypotension
Weak pulse
Weakness
Skin findings (pallor, sweating)
Fatigue

Signs and Symptoms of Pulmonary Congestion	Tachypnea Labored respirations Jugular venous distention Frothy sputum Cyanosis Dyspnea
Causes of Primary Pump Problems	Myocardial Infarction Drug overdose/poisoning
Secondary Pump Problems	As oxygen, glucose and ATP (adenosine triphosphate) are depleted, essentially all patients in shock will eventually develop a secondary pump problem

Therapy –
Overview

Patients in pump failure may require:

- Treatment of a coexisting rate or volume problem
- Correction of underlying problems (hypoglycemia, hypoxia, drug overdose, poisoning)
- Support for failing pump
  - Agents to increase contractility (dopamine, dobutamine, etc.)
  - Vasodilators to decrease afterload
  - Vasodilators, diuretics to decrease preload
  - Mechanical assistance (intra-aortic balloon pump)
  - Surgery (coronary artery bypass grafts, valves, heart transplant)

Systolic BP
< 70 mm Hg
with signs of shock

Very high mortality

Often a result of a pump AND volume problem

1. If pulmonary edema absent, administer fluid challenge of 250-500 ml of normal saline to assure adequate ventricular filling pressure
2. Administer norepinephrine infusion (0.5-30 μg/min) until systolic BP 70-100 mm Hg
   - Norepinephrine has both inotropic (β-1) and vasoconstrictive (α) properties
3. Once BP increased to 70-100 mm Hg, attempt to switch to an infusion of dopamine (2.5-20 μg/kg/min)
4. Mobilize balloon pump team and alert cath lab if associated with acute MI
5. If acute MI and pump failure, consider transfer to facility capable of catheterization, angioplasty and cardiovascular surgery

Systolic BP 70-100 mm Hg with signs of shock	1. If pulmonary edema absent, administer fluid challenge of 250-500 ml of normal saline to assure adequate ventricular filling pressure 2. Dopamine is usually the drug of choice with systolic BP of 70-100 mm Hg • Start at 2.5 μg/kg/min and titrate to a maximum of 20 μg/kg/min • If > 20 μg/kg/min of dopamine needed, consider adding norepinephrine (has fewer chronotropic effects)
Systolic BP > 100 mm Hg and normal diastolic BP with signs of shock	Dobutamine drug of choice when BP in this range • Start dobutamine at 2 μg/kg/min and titrate to maximum of 20 μg/kg/min • Once dobutamine started, begin decreasing dopamine infusion
Diastolic BP > 110 mm Hg with signs of shock	Pump failure and diastolic hypertension usually associated with pulmonary congestion and edema • In the absence of ischemia, nitroprusside (0.1-5.0 μg/kg/min) is the drug of choice (> afterload reduction than nitroglycerin) • If ischemia present, IV nitroglycerin (10-20 μg/min) preferred

ACUTE MYOCARDIAL INFARCTION WITH PULMONARY EDEMA

First-line Actions

1. Sitting position with feet dependent
   • Increases lung volume and vital capacity
   • Decreases work of respiration
   • Decreases venous return to the heart
2. High flow O_2
3. Intubate as needed
4. Furosemide IV 0.5-1.0 mg/kg
   • If the patient is already taking oral furosemide, initial dose is usually twice the daily oral dose
5. Morphine IV 1-3 mg
6. Sublingual nitroglycerin if BP near normal

Second-line Actions

1. Nitroglycerin IV (if BP > 100)
2. Nitroprusside IV (if pressure too high)
3. Dopamine IV 2.5-20 μg/kg/min (if BP < 100)
4. Dobutamine IV (normotensive pump failure)

Third-line Actions

- Patients with pump failure and acute pulmonary edema resistant to previous actions
- Require invasive hemodynamic monitoring in an ICU or specialized tertiary care facility

1. Amrinone (0.75 mg/kg over 2-3 minutes followed by 5-15 μg/kg/min)
   - Inotropic and vasodilatory effects similar to dobutamine
2. Aminophylline (5 mg/kg over 10-20 minutes followed by 0.5-0.7 mg/kg/hr)
   - May be effective in patients with acute bronchospasm ("cardiac asthma")
   - Should be reserved for severe bronchospasm
   - Avoid in patients with supraventricular dysrhythmias, with ischemic heart disease
3. Thrombolytic therapy of limited value in patients with acute MI and pump failure
4. Angioplasty may be of benefit if performed within 18 hours of symptom onset
5. Intra-aortic balloon pump ("bridge" until surgery)
6. Surgical intervention (coronary artery bypass grafting, valve repair, heart transplant)

ACUTE MYOCARDIAL INFARCTION WITH HYPERTENSION

Definition and Significance

1. Hypertension = systolic BP > than 140 mm Hg, diastolic BP > than 90 mm Hg
2. Potentially harmful in acute MI
   - May increase myocardial oxygen demand
   - May exacerbate ischemia or infarction
3. Precautions
   - Hypertension may be transient
   - Overtreatment $\rightarrow$ severe hypotension

Therapy

1. Relief of pain and anxiety
   - Oxygen
   - Sublingual nitroglycerin
   - Morphine

2. If pulmonary congestion present:
   - IV furosemide

3. If unresponsive to initial therapy
   - IV nitroglycerin (especially if CHF present)
   - β-blockers in tachycardia and high cardiac output
   - Consider IV nitroprusside

REFERENCES

1. Bayer AJ, Chadha J.S., Farag RR, Pathy MS. Changing presentation of myocardial infarction with increasing age. *J of the Am Geri Soc* 34:263, 1986.

2. Fesmire FM, Smith EE. Continuous 12-lead electrocardiograph monitoring in the emergency department. *Am J Emerg Med* 11:54-60, 1993.

3. Emergency Cardiac Care Committee and Subcommittees, American Heart Association. Guidelines for cardiopulmonary resuscitation and emergency cardiac care. *JAMA* 268:2199, 1992.

4. Weaver WD, Eisenberg MS, Martin JS, Litwin PE, Shaeffer SM, Ho MT, Kudenshuk P, Hallstrom AP, Cerqueira MD, Copass MK, Kennedy JW, Cobb LA, Ritchie JL: Myocardial infarction triage and intervention project - phase I: patient characteristics and feasibility of prehospital thrombolytic therapy. *J Am Coll Cardiol* 15:925-931, 1990.

5. Wilcox RG, von der Lippe G, Olsson CG, Jensen G, Skene AM, Hampton JR: Trial of tissue plasminogen activator for mortality reduction in acute myocardial infarction: Anglo-Scandinavian study of early thrombolysis (ASSET), *Lancet* 2:525-530, 1988.

6. Wesley RC, Resh W, Zimmerman D: Reconsiderations of the routine and preferential use of lidocaine in the emergent treatment of ventricular arrhythmias, *Critical Care Med* 19:1439-1444, 1991.

7. Emergency Cardiac Care Committee and Subcommittees, American Heart Association. Guidelines for cardiopulmonary resuscitation and emergency cardiac care. *JAMA* 268:2225, 1992.

8. Emergency Cardiac Care Committee and Subcommittees, American Heart Association. Guidelines for cardiopulmonary resuscitation and emergency cardiac care. *JAMA* 268:2217, 1992.

9. Emergency Cardiac Care Committee and Subcommittees, American Heart Association. Guidelines for cardiopulmonary resuscitation and emergency cardiac care. *JAMA* 268:2227, 1992.

ACLS/MYOCARDIAL INFARCTION QUIZ

1. In an adult victim cardiac arrest, the bystander should:

    a. activate the EMS system after 1 minute of rescue efforts
    b. determine unresponsiveness, activate the EMS system and then initiate CPR
    c. assess the pulse, assess breathing, open the airway and then activate the EMS system
    d. open the airway, assess breathing, ventilate, assess the pulse, and then activate the EMS system

2. Which of the following is NOT one of the links in the chain of survival?

    a. early CPR
    b. early warning
    c. early access
    d. early defibrillation

3. Cardiopulmonary-cerebral resuscitation (CPCR):

    a. is a term that is synonymous with acute myocardial infarction
    b. is a term used to emphasize the need to preserve the cerebral viability of the cardiac arrest victim
    c. is a term that refers to gradual circulatory failure and collapse of circulation before loss of pulse
    d. is a term that refers to an abrupt loss of consciousness and pulse without prior circulatory collapse

4. Which of the following statements regarding the chain of survival is INCORRECT?

    a. bystander CPR frequently causes significant injury to victims
    b. the AHA recommends AEDs be placed in gathering places of more than 10,000 people
    c. in addition to defibrillation, intubation and IV medications may significantly improve the outcome of the cardiac arrest patient
    d. the goal of every EMS system should be to attain a two ACLS and two BLS emergency medical services provider level of response

5. The greatest risk of death from heart attack occurs:

    a. within the first 2 hours after the onset of symptoms
    b. between 3 and 8 hours after the onset of symptoms
    c. between 10 and 24 hours after the onset of symptoms
    d. between 24 and 48 hours after the onset of symptoms

6. The term "second-degree AV block, type I" is synonymous with:

   a. Mobitz II

   b. AV dissociation

   c. Mobitz I or Wenckebach

   d. Mobitz II or Wenckebach

7. Medications which may be used in the management of ventricular fibrillation include:

   1. bretylium

   2. epinephrine

   3. adenosine

   4. lidocaine

   5. magnesium sulfate

   a. 2, 3

   b. 1, 2, 4

   c. 2, 4, 5

   d. 1, 2, 4, 5

8. The initial recommended adult IV dose of epinephrine administered in cardiac arrest is:

   a. 1.0 mg IV bolus

   b. 0.5-1.0 mg IV bolus

   c. 1-1.5 mg/kg IV bolus

   d. 5 mg/kg continuous IV infusion

9. A 57 year old male is complaining of chest pain and difficulty breathing. He is disoriented and extremely anxious. Examination reveals bibasilar crackles; a weak and irregular carotid pulse and a blood pressure of 60/30. The cardiac monitor displays atrial fibrillation at a rate of 150-190 beats/minute. Management of this patient should include:

   a. administration of sublingual nitroglycerin for pain relief

   b. administration of 6 mg of adenosine rapid IV bolus and reassessment of the patient

   c. administration of 2.5 mg of verapamil slow IV bolus and reassessment of the patient

   d. administration of sedation, performing synchronized countershock at 100J and reassessment of the patient

10. The link in the chain of survival most likely to improve survival is:

    a. early CPR

    b. early ACLS

    c. early access

    d. early defibrillation

11. Emergency departments should take no more than ___ to assess and begin thrombolytic treatment for patients with evidence of coronary thrombosis and no reasons for exclusion.

    a. 1-2 hours

    b. 2-4 hours

    c. 30-60 minutes

    d. 10-15 minutes

12. A 62 year old male is complaining of excruciating chest pain radiating to his left arm and jaw. He states the pain has been present for the past hour and is unrelieved with rest. His blood pressure is 134/62, respiratory rate 16. He is warm, diaphoretic and anxious. The cardiac monitor shows a sinus rhythm at 80 beats/minute without ectopy. Which of the following most correctly reflects the recommended treatment sequence for this patient?

    a. oxygen, dopamine infusion at 5-20 µg/kg/min

    b. oxygen, epinephrine 1 mg IV bolus every 3-5 minutes

    c. assess ABCs, CPR until a defibrillator is available then defibrillation with 200J

    d. oxygen, nitroglycerin, pain relief with narcotics, aspirin, and thrombolytic therapy if no reason for exclusion

13. Sodium bicarbonate is considered a Class I (definitely helpful) intervention in:

    a. hypoxic lactic acidosis

    b. known preexisting hyperkalemia

    c. overdose due to cyclic antidepressants

    d. upon return of spontaneous circulation after a long arrest interval

14. In which of the following situations would an epinephrine bolus be indicated?

    a. atrial fibrillation

    b. sinus bradycardia

    c. acute pulmonary edema

    d. pulseless electrical activity

15. Potential causes of pulseless electrical activity include all of the following EXCEPT:
    a. severe acidosis
    b. cardiac tamponade
    c. massive pulmonary embolism
    d. chronic obstructive pulmonary disease

16. A 72 year old male is complaining of severe substernal chest pain. He is awake, pale and diaphoretic. BP 110/64, P 190, R 16. The cardiac monitor shows ventricular tachycardia. Recommended treatment guidelines include:
    a. initiate CPR, defibrillate with 200J
    b. O_2, IV, sublingual nitroglycerin, adenosine 6 mg rapid IV push
    c. O_2, IV, consider medications; if unsuccessful and the patient's condition is unchanged, sedate and perform synchronized countershock with 100J
    d. O_2, IV, consider medications; if unsuccessful and the patient's condition is unchanged, sedate and perform unsynchronized countershock with 200J

17. Control of chest pain in the patient having a myocardial infarction is important for all of the following reasons EXCEPT:
    a. relief of pain usually relieves anxiety
    b. relief of pain may decrease the risk of dysrhythmias
    c. relief of pain results in increased myocardial oxygen demand
    d. pain releases catecholamines and may increase myocardial damage

18. A 56 year old female is complaining of "palpitations." When questioned, she denies chest pain or shortness of breath. Her blood pressure is 134/82, pulse 180, respirations 18. The cardiac monitor shows a narrow-QRS tachycardia without visible P waves. Recommended treatment for this patient includes:
    a. O_2, IV, vagal maneuvers, adenosine 6 mg rapid IV bolus
    b. O_2, IV, vagal maneuvers, verapamil 2.5 mg slow IV bolus
    c. O_2, IV, atropine 1.0 mg IV every 3-5 minutes to a maximum of 3 mg
    d. O_2, IV, sedate and perform synchronized countershock with 50J

19. A 55 year old female has arrived in the Emergency Department complaining of severe chest pain. Her blood pressure is 126/72, pulse 138, respirations 14. The cardiac monitor shows a sinus tachycardia without ectopy. Management of this patient should include:
    a. O_2, IV, nitroglycerin, morphine
    b. O_2, IV, verapamil 2.5 mg slow IV bolus
    c. O_2, IV, nitroglycerin, morphine, lidocaine
    d. O_2, IV, vagal maneuvers, adenosine 6 mg rapid IV bolus

20. Atropine may be useful in treating all of the following EXCEPT:

    a. asystole
    b. symptomatic sinus bradycardia
    c. paroxysmal supraventricular tachycardia
    d. bradycardic pulseless electrical activity

21. Lidocaine is indicated in all of the following situations EXCEPT:

    a. narrow-complex supraventricular tachycardia
    b. wide-complex tachycardia of uncertain origin
    c. ventricular tachycardia with a pulse
    d. VT and VF that persist after defibrillation and administration of epinephrine

22. The recommended IV dose of morphine sulfate is:

    a. 1-1.5 mg/kg every 5-10 minutes
    b. 1-3 mg every 5 minutes, titrated to desired response
    c. 6 mg repeated every 1-2 minutes to a maximum dose of 30 mg
    d. 5 mg/kg repeated every 5 minutes, titrated to desired response

23. VF/VT is termed "refractory" or "persistent" after:

    a. basic CPR, intubation, ventilation, and an initial defibrillation at 200 joules
    b. basic CPR, intubation, ventilation, and defibrillation with three "stacked shocks"
    c. basic CPR, intubation, ventilation, and defibrillation with three "stacked shocks" and an initial bolus of epinephrine
    d. basic CPR, intubation, ventilation, four defibrillations and one or more doses of epinephrine

24. First-line actions in the treatment of the normotensive patient with acute pulmonary edema include:

    a. oxygen, nitroprusside, dopamine
    b. oxygen, amrinone, aminophylline and thrombolytic therapy
    c. oxygen, furosemide, sublingual nitroglycerin, and morphine
    d. oxygen, dobutamine, furosemide, morphine and aminophylline

25. A 47 year old male is complaining of crushing midsternal pain, dizziness and nausea. His blood pressure is 74/40, pulse 48, respirations 16. The cardiac monitor displays a Second Degree AV Block, Type I. Recommended treatment guidelines for this patient would include:

a. ABCs, O_2, IV, adenosine 6 mg rapid IV push
b. ABCs, O_2, IV, sublingual nitroglycerin, transcutaneous pacing
c. ABCs, O_2, IV, atropine 0.5-1 mg IV every 3-5 minutes to a maximum of 2-3 mg
d. ABCs, O_2, IV, morphine 1-3 mg titrated to pain relief, lidocaine 1-1.5 mg/kg

ACLS/MYOCARDIAL INFARCTION QUIZ ANSWER SHEET

1. A   B   C   D
2. A   B   C   D
3. A   B   C   D
4. A   B   C   D
5. A   B   C   D
6. A   B   C   D
7. A   B   C   D
8. A   B   C   D
9. A   B   C   D
10. A   B   C   D
11. A   B   C   D
12. A   B   C   D
13. A   B   C   D
14. A   B   C   D
15. A   B   C   D
16. A   B   C   D
17. A   B   C   D
18. A   B   C   D
19. A   B   C   D
20. A   B   C   D
21. A   B   C   D
22. A   B   C   D
23. A   B   C   D
24. A   B   C   D
25. A   B   C   D

ACLS/MYOCARDIAL INFARCTION QUIZ ANSWERS

QUESTION	ANSWER	RATIONALE	JAMA PAGE REFERENCE
1	B	Early CPR, combined with early activation of the EMS system (thus earlier access to defibrillation), is the key to optimal survival.	2184, 2291
2	B	The links in the chain of survival are early access, early CPR, early defibrillation and early ACLS.	2176
3	B	Cardiopulmonary-cerebral resuscitation (CPCR) is a term used to emphasize the need to preserve the cerebral viability of the cardiac arrest victim.	2176
4	A	"Bystander CPR rarely causes significant injury to victims, even when started inappropriately on people not in cardiac arrest."	2291
5	A	The greatest risk of death from heart attack occurs within the first 2 hours after the onset of symptoms.	2177
6	C	Second degree AV block, type I is current terminology used to describe Wenckebach or Mobitz I.	N/A
7	D	Medications used in the management of VF include epinephrine, lidocaine, bretylium, magnesium sulfate, procainamide and, possibly, sodium bicarbonate. Adenosine is not indicated in the management of VF.	2217
8	A	The recommended initial adult dose of epinephrine in cardiac arrest is 1 mg IV.	2218
9	D	This patient is unstable (chest pain, altered level of consciousness, hypotension, difficulty breathing). Administer sedation and perform synchronized countershock with 100J and reassess the patient. "If the patient experiences serious signs and symptoms, clinicians should prepare for immediate cardioversion."	2224

10	D	Early defibrillation is the link in the chain of survival most likely to improve survival.	2291
11	C	The "door to drug" interval is 30 to 60 min to assess and begin thrombolytic therapy.	2230
12	D	Oxygen, nitroglycerin, pain relief with narcotics, aspirin, and thrombolytic therapy (if no reason for exclusion) are all treatments to consider for the patient suspected of experiencing an acute MI.	2230
13	B	Sodium bicarbonate is considered Class I (definitely helpful) in known preexisting hyperkalemia; Class IIa (probably helpful) in overdose due to cyclic antidepressants; Class IIb upon return of spontaneous circulation after a long arrest interval; and a Class III (may be harmful) intervention in hypoxic lactic acidosis.	2219
14	D	An epinephrine bolus is indicated in the management of pulseless electrical activity, pulseless VT or VF and asystole.	2219
15	D	Potential causes of pulseless electrical activity include: (MATCHx4ED) → myocardial infarction (massive), acidosis, tension pneumothorax, cardiac tamponade, hypovolemia, hypoxia, hyperkalemia, hypothermia, embolism (massive pulmonary) and drug overdose	2219
16	C	O_2, IV, consider medications; if unsuccessful and the patient's condition is unchanged, sedate and perform synchronized countershock with 100J.	2222-2223
17	C	Relief of pain is a high priority in the management of the patient experiencing an acute MI. Pain relief may decrease the incidence of dysrhythmias, decrease anxiety and decrease myocardial oxygen demand. It is thought that the presence of pain causes a release of catecholamines which result in increased myocardial damage.	2230

18	A	This patient is clinically stable. Administer oxygen, initiate an IV, attempt vagal maneuvers, and, if unsuccessful, administer adenosine 6 mg rapid IV bolus. Repeat with 12 mg of adenosine in 1-2 minutes if necessary.	2223
19	A	O_2, IV, nitroglycerin, morphine. Routine prophylactic use of lidocaine is no longer recommended.	2230-2231
20	C	Atropine is useful in the management of asystole and pulseless electrical activity with a bradycardic rhythm. It is also useful in symptomatic patients whose ECG displays a narrow-QRS bradycardia (sinus bradycardia, junctional escape rhythm, second degree AV block, type I and third-degree AV block with a narrow-QRS).	2207, 2222
21	A	Lidocaine is not indicated in the treatment of narrow-complex SVT.	2206, 2223
22	B	The recommended dose of morphine sulfate is 1-3 mg every 5 minutes, titrated to desired response.	2206
23	D	VF/VT is considered "refractory" or "persistent" after basic CPR, intubation, ventilation, four defibrillations and one or more doses of epinephrine	2218
24	C	Oxygen, furosemide, sublingual nitroglycerin, and morphine are first-line actions in the management of the normotensive patient with acute pulmonary edema.	2227, 2229
25	C	Management of this patient should include evaluation of the ABCs, O_2, IV, and atropine 0.5-1 mg IV q 3-5 minutes to a maximum of 2-3 mg. Atropine is considered a Class IIa (probably helpful) intervention in the management of AV block at the nodal level.	2207, 2222

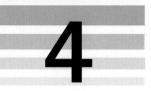

4 Airway Adjuncts

Objectives:

Upon completion of this chapter, you will be able to:

1. Describe the head-tilt/chin-lift and jaw-thrust methods for opening the airway.

2. Describe the method of correct sizing, insertion technique and possible complications associated with insertion of the oropharyngeal airway and nasopharyngeal airway.

3. Describe the indications, insertion technique and possible complications associated with insertion of an esophageal obturator or esophageal gastric tube airway.

4. Describe the oxygen liter flow per minute and estimated oxygen percentage delivered for each of the following devices:
   - Nasal cannula
   - Simple face mask
   - Venturi mask
   - Pocket mask
   - Nonrebreather mask
   - Bag-valve-device

5. Identify the desirable features of the bag-valve device.

6. Describe the advantages and disadvantages associated with the use of the bag-valve device.

7. Identify the recommended tidal volume that should be delivered when using the bag-valve device.

8. Describe the indications, advantages and technique for performing endotracheal intubation.

9. Describe the technique for confirming proper placement of an esophageal obturator airway and endotracheal tube.

10. Describe advantages and disadvantages associated with the use of automatic transport ventilators.

11. Describe the indications, complications and techniques for performing transtracheal ventilation and surgical cricothyrotomy.

12. Describe correct suctioning technique and complications associated with this procedure.

HEAD AND JAW POSITION

Head-Tilt/Chin-Lift

- The patient's head is tilted back by placing one hand on the forehead and the fingers of the other hand under the patient's chin.
- Should NOT be used if cervical spine injury is suspected.

Jaw-Thrust

- The angles of the patient's lower jaw are grasped with both hands, one on each side, displacing the mandible forward.
- Should be used to open the airway when cervical spine injury is suspected.

OROPHARYNGEAL AIRWAY (OPA)

Description and Function

Class I - Definitely helpful

1. Semicircular shaped plastic device that is placed on top of the tongue
2. When correctly positioned, the distal tip will lie between the base of the tongue and the back of the throat to prevent the tongue from occluding the airway, allowing ventilation to occur

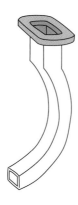

Figure 4-1   The oropharyngeal airway.

Adult Sizes

1. Size determined by aligning the airway on the side of the patient's face and selecting an airway that extends from the earlobe to the corner of the mouth
2. Size of the airway based on the distance, in millimeters, from the flange to the distal tip
3. Recommended sizes:
   - Large adult = 100 mm (size 5)
   - Medium adult = 90 mm (size 4)
   - Small adult = 80 mm (size 3)

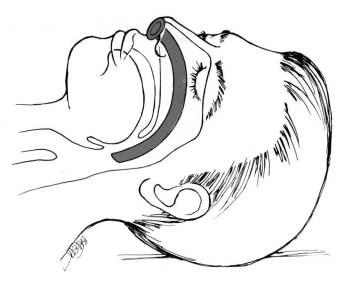

Figure 4-4   Nasopharyngeal airway in correct position.

Complications	1. Avoid forceful insertion as it may cause abrasions or lacerations of the nasal mucosa and result in significant bleeding
	2. If the tube is too long, it may enter the esophagus, causing gastric distention and hypoventilation
	3. Most conscious and semiconscious patients can tolerate this airway but the gag reflex may be stimulated in sensitive patients, precipitating laryngospasm and vomiting.

NASAL CANNULA (NASAL PRONGS)

Description and Function

1. Piece of plastic tubing with two ports designed to deliver supplemental oxygen through the nares

2. Can deliver oxygen concentrations of 25-45% at 1-6 liters/min flow

    Formula = 21% (room air) + (4 × O_2 flow in liters/minute)

    1 liter/minute   = 25%
    2 liters/minute = 29%
    3 liters/minute = 33%
    4 liters/minute = 37%
    5 liters/minute = 41%
    6 liters/minute = 45%

Advantages

1. Well tolerated by most patients

2. No rebreathing of expired air

3. Particularly valuable in patients with COPD for whom low O_2 concentrations are desirable

Disadvantages

1. Can only be used in the spontaneously breathing patient

2. When higher concentrations of O_2 are needed, preferable devices include the nonrebreather mask (Venturi mask for COPD patients)

3. Actual amount of inspired O_2 depends on respiratory rate and depth

SIMPLE FACE MASK (STANDARD MASK)

Description and Function

1. Plastic device with several small holes on each side that allows for inhalation and exhalation of air. There is also a port for delivery of supplemental O_2 on the lower portion of the mask.
   - Air holes on the sides of the mask allow passage of inspired AND expired air
   - Supplemental oxygen is directed into the mask
   - Concentration of inspired oxygen less than that with nonrebreather mask because the supplemental O_2 mixes with room air
2. The O_2 flow rate must be higher than 5 liters/minute to avoid the accumulation of exhaled air in the mask reservoir that might be rebreathed.
3. Recommended flow rate is 8-10 liters/minute. At this flow rate, the device provides approximately 40-60% oxygen.

Advantages

Higher O_2 concentration delivered than by nasal cannula

Disadvantages

1. Variability in actual inspired O_2 concentration (this is because the amount of air that mixes with supplemental O_2 is dependent on the patient's inspiratory flow rate)
2. Because of the variability in delivered FiO_2 with this mask, a nonrebreather mask may be preferable when high concentrations of O_2 are required
3. Not tolerated well in severely dyspneic patients
4. Can only be used with spontaneously breathing patients

VENTURI MASK

Description and Function

Similar in concept to the simple face mask with a modification that allows relatively fixed concentrations of supplemental O_2 to be inspired

Advantages

1. Greater control of the O_2 concentration administered
2. Preferred in COPD patients because it provides precise O_2 concentrations

Disadvantages

1. Can only be used with spontaneously breathing patients
2. Uncomfortable for prolonged use

NONREBREATHER MASK

Description and
Function

Adjunct of choice when high concentrations of O_2 are needed in the spontaneously breathing patient because it can consistently deliver an FiO_2 of up to 100% at 10-15 liters/minute flow.

1. One-way valve present on each side of the nonrebreather mask that allows exhaled air to escape but prevents room air from being inspired
2. Supplemental oxygen is directed into the reservoir bag of the nonrebreather device
3. The patient inhales 100% oxygen from the reservoir because the one-way valve prevents exhaled air from entering the reservoir bag
4. At 10-15 liters/minute the O_2 concentration is almost 100%.

Advantages

Higher oxygen concentration delivered than with nasal cannula or simple face mask

Disadvantages

1. Mask must fit snugly on the patient's face to prevent room air from mixing with O_2 inhaled from the reservoir bag
2. Can only be used with spontaneously breathing patients

Special
Considerations

1. The reservoir bag must remain completely inflated when using this device so sufficient supplemental O_2 is available for each breath
2. Must use high flow rates of 10-15 liters/minute

POCKET MASK

Description and
Function

1. Similar to the mask used with bag-valve devices with an additional port through which supplemental O_2 can be administered
2. Inspired O_2 concentrations:
   Exhaled air (mouth-to-mask) = 16-17%
   Room air = 21%
   10 liters/minute = 50%
   15 liters/minute = 80%
   30 liters/minute = 100%

Desirable Mask Features

1. Transparent material to allow detection of regurgitation
2. Capable of a tight fit on the face with an O_2 inlet of standard 15-mm/22-mm coupling size
3. Available in one average size for adults with additional sizes for infants and children
4. Should be equipped with a one-way valve that diverts the victim's exhaled gas when used for mouth-to-mask ventilation

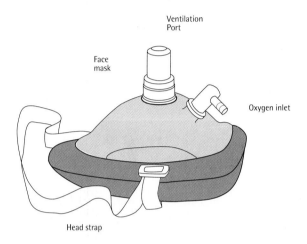

Ventilation Port

Face mask

Oxygen inlet

Head strap

Figure 4-5. The pocket mask.

Application

1. Rescuer positions self at head of patient
2. The mask is placed on the patient's face and secured with both hands
   a. The thumbs stabilize the mask across the bridge of the nose
   b. Upward pressure is applied to the mandible just in front of the earlobes using the remaining fingers of both hands while maintaining proper head position
3. The rescuer blows through the port of the mask observing the rise and fall of the chest

Advantages

1. Eliminates need for direct mouth-to-mouth contact between patient and rescuer
2. Administration of supplemental O_2 possible
3. Eliminates exposure to exhaled air
4. Easy to teach and learn
5. Provides effective ventilation and oxygenation
6. Aesthetically more acceptable than mouth-to-mouth
7. May be used on the apneic patient as well as the spontaneously breathing patient
8. *Mouth-to-mask ventilation can deliver a higher tidal volume than a bag-valve-mask device in the nonintubated patient (manikin studies)*

Disadvantages

Rescuer fatigue

BAG-VALVE DEVICES

Description and
Function

Consists of a self-inflating bag and a nonrebreathing valve with an adapter that can be attached to a mask, endotracheal tube or other invasive airway device

Desirable Features

1. Self-refilling bag that is easily cleaned and sterilized
2. Nonjam valve system allowing for a minimum oxygen inlet flow of 15 L/min
3. No pop-off (pressure-release) valve
   - To properly ventilate patients in cardiac arrest, much higher than usual airway pressures are often needed
   - Pop-off valves may prevent generation of sufficient peak airway pressure to overcome the increase in airway resistance
4. A clear mask
5. A system for delivering high concentrations of O_2 through an ancillary oxygen inlet at the back of the bag or by an oxygen reservoir
6. A true nonrebreathing valve
7. Must perform satisfactorily under all common environmental conditions and extremes of temperature
8. Available in both adult and pediatric sizes

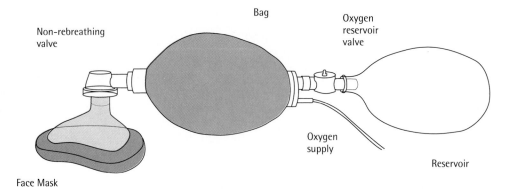

Figure 4-6   The bag-valve device.

Oxygen Delivery

BVM without supplemental oxygen = 21% (room air)
BVM at 12-15 L/min O_2 without reservoir = 40-60%
BVM at 12-15 L/min O_2 and reservoir = 90-100%

Tidal volume delivered should be 10-15 ml/kg
- Slightly more volume may be needed for the very obese patient
- Slightly less volume may be needed for patients with fragile intrathoracic airways or diminished lung volumes

Advantages

1. Immediate ventilation of patient with oxygen enriched mixture
2. Sense of compliance of lungs is conveyed to operator
   - *Compliance* refers to the resistance of the patient's lung tissue to ventilation. For example, lung compliance is decreased in tension pneumothorax resulting in increased resistance (poor compliance); harder to ventilate the patient.
3. Increased oxygen delivery to the patient
4. Can be used with the spontaneously breathing patient as well as the apneic patient

Disadvantages

1. Most frequent problem with the bag-valve device is the inability to provide adequate ventilatory volume due to the difficulty in providing a leakproof seal to the face while simultaneously maintaining an open airway
2. Should only be used by trained operators (ideally a two- rescuer operation - one to hold the mask to the face and maintain an open airway, the other to compress the bag with both hands)
3. Gastric distention
4. Difficult to use by inexperienced operators

OXYGEN-POWERED MANUALLY TRIGGERED DEVICES (DEMAND-VALVE RESUSCITATOR)

Description

1. Allows positive-pressure ventilation with 100% oxygen
2. Can be attached to a face mask, endotracheal tube, EOA, EGTA or tracheostomy tube
3. Consists of a high-pressure tubing connecting the oxygen supply and a valve that is activated by a lever or push button; when the valve is open, oxygen flows into the patient

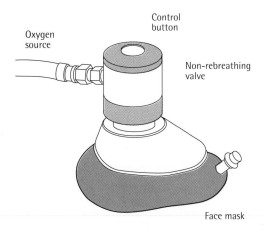

Figure 4-7 Oxygen-powered breathing device.

Complications	1. Gastric distention
	2. Barotrauma to the lungs
	• Pneumothorax
	• Subcutaneous emphysema
Contraindications	Not for use in pediatric patients

AUTOMATIC TRANSPORT VENTILATORS (ATVs)

Class I - Definitely helpful

Advantages

1. Frees the rescuer for other tasks when used in intubated patients
2. In nonintubated patients, the rescuer has both hands free for mask and airway maintenance
3. Cricoid pressure can be applied with one hand while the other seals the mask on the face
4. Once set, provide a specific tidal volume, respiratory rate and minute ventilation
5. Improved lung inflation with diminished or absent gastric insufflation compared to mouth-to-mask, bag-valve-mask and manually triggered devices due to the lower inspiratory flow rates and longer inspiratory times provided by ATVs

Disadvantages

1. Require an oxygen source (or, sometimes, electric power)
2. Many ATVs should not be used in children < five years of age

SUCTION DEVICES

Description and Function

1. Whistle-Tip Catheter
   - Used to clear blood or mucus from an endotracheal tube or the nasopharynx
2. Rigid Pharyngeal Suction (Tonsil-tip, Yankauer)
   - Used to clear secretions, blood clots and other foreign material from the mouth and pharynx

Technique

1. Hyperventilate before suctioning
2. Insert catheter WITHOUT applying suction
3. Apply intermittent suction by closing the side opening while withdrawing the catheter in a rotating motion
4. Suction should not be applied for more than 10 seconds
5. Before repeating the procedure, hyperventilate the patient

Complications

1. Severe hypoxia
2. May trigger coughing, resulting in increased intracranial pressure and a reduction in cerebral blood flow
3. Damage to the mucosa → edema, hemorrhage, ulcerated areas that may result in tracheal infection
4. Increased arterial pressure and tachycardia
5. Bradycardia and hypotension due to vagal stimulation

ESOPHAGEAL OBTURATOR AIRWAY (EOA)

Class IIb - POSSIBLY helpful

Description and Function

1. Tube 37 cm in length; open at the top, closed (blind) tip on the distal end
2. Inflation of the cuff just above the closed end occludes the esophagus (30-35 ml of air)
3. Small side holes present on the upper third of the tube. When the EOA has been correctly placed, the holes lie at the level of the posterior pharynx
   - Air enters through the upper end of the EOA and exits through the side holes into the pharynx → enters the trachea→ inflates the lungs because the esophagus is occluded and the face mask is appropriately applied to maintain a good seal

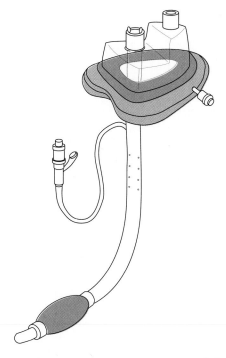

Figure 4-8   The esophageal obturator airway (EOA).

Indications

Unconscious and apneic adult patient

Insertion

1. Attach the tube to the mask and test the cuff for leaks

2. Deflate the cuff and lubricate the tube

3. Hyperventilate with 100% oxygen

4. With the head in a NEUTRAL position, elevate the tongue and jaw with one gloved hand while inserting the tube through the mouth into the esophagus until the mask rests on the face to assure the cuff will lie below the level of the carina

   • The carina is the point where the trachea bifurcates into the right and left mainstem bronchi (approximately the level of the 5th or 6th thoracic vertebrae)

5. Deliver several positive pressure ventilations to assess tube position (observe chest rise)

6. Auscultate breath sounds

   • Listen in the apices and lateral lungs fields (midaxillary line) and observe chest rise

   • Listen over the epigastrium - gurgling suggests the tube has been improperly placed into the trachea (balloon is occluding the trachea and air is entering the esophagus)

7. Once proper tube placement is confirmed, inflate the EOA cuff with 30-35 ml of air and disconnect the syringe

8. Continue ventilation of the patient

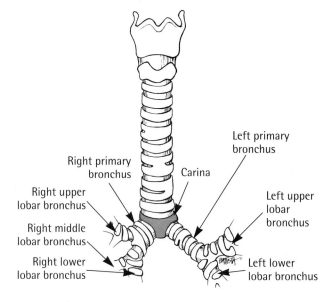

Figure 4-9   The carina is the point where the trachea bifurcates into the right and left mainstem bronchi.

Advantages

1. Visualization not required for insertion

   • Thought to be more quickly and easily inserted than an endotracheal tube

2. Reasonable technique for use in suspected neck injury since the head does not need to be hyperextended

Disadvantages	1. Inadequate tidal volumes due to face mask leak
	2. Inadvertent tracheal intubation
	3. Esophageal laceration and rupture
	4. High incidence of regurgitation on removal of the tube, increased risk of aspiration

Disadvantages

1. Inadequate tidal volumes due to face mask leak
2. Inadvertent tracheal intubation
3. Esophageal laceration and rupture
4. High incidence of regurgitation on removal of the tube, increased risk of aspiration

Contraindications

1. Should not be used in conscious patients
2. Should not be used in children under 16 (is only available in one size)
3. Should not be used in cases of known esophageal disease
4. Should not be used for more than two hours
5. Should not be used when caustic substances have been ingested

Removal

1. Endotracheal tube securely in place
2. Awake patient turned on his/her side
3. Suction available
4. Deflate cuff and remove tube
5. Suction!!

ESOPHAGEAL GASTRIC TUBE AIRWAY (EGTA)

Class IIb - POSSIBLY helpful

Description and Function

1. Improved version of the EOA
   - Route for gastric decompression added
   - Reduces the chance for regurgitation and aspiration
2. Distal end of tube is open, allowing passage of a tube for gastric decompression
3. EGTA added a second port on the mask for ventilation and removed the small holes that are present on the upper half of the EOA

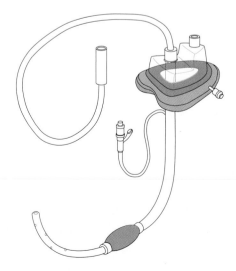

Figure 4-10   The esophageal gastric tube airway (EGTA).

PHARYNGOTRACHEAL LUMEN AIRWAY (PTLA)

Class IIb - POSSIBLY helpful

Description and
Function

- Double-lumen tube allowing either tracheal or esophageal placement
- Was developed to address the problems with EOA use (inadvertent tracheal intubation and proper face-to-mask seal)
- Blind insertion technique

Consists of two tubes, each having an internal diameter of 8 mm

1. First tube green in color at the proximal end
   - Short, wide tube (21 cm)
   - Balloon located at proximal portion of tube which seals off the oropharynx when inflated
   - Air entering the tube at the proximal end enters the pharynx
2. Second tube clear in color at the proximal end
   - May be inserted into either the trachea or esophagus
   - Smaller, distal balloon inflated and seals off either the trachea or esophagus
   - When this tube is in the esophagus, the patient is ventilated through the first tube (functions as an EOA)
   - When this tube is positioned in the trachea, the patient is ventilated directly through it (functions as a standard endotracheal tube)
3. Slide clamp allows the oropharyngeal cuff to be deflated and the small, distal balloon to remain inflated when intubating around the PtLA
4. Adjustable cloth neck strap holds the PtLA in place

Advantages

1. Visualization not required for insertion
2. Reasonable technique for use in suspected neck injury since the head does not need to be hyperextended
3. Because of the oropharyngeal balloon, need for a face mask is eliminated

Disadvantages

1. Reports of inadequate seal with the pharyngeal balloon
2. Design of the device may pose a problem when attempting to replace the PtLA with a tracheal tube

Indications

1. Inability of the rescuer to ventilate the unconscious patient with conventional methods

2. Inability of the patient to protect his/her own airway (coma, areflexia, cardiac arrest)

3. Cardiac arrest with ongoing chest compressions

   - *Once an ET tube is in place, ventilation does not need to be synchronized with chest compressions. Ventilations should be delivered asynchronously at a rate of 12-15 per minute*

4. Inability of the conscious patient to ventilate adequately

Technique

1. Check the endotracheal tube cuff for leaks (must be tested before insertion)

2. A stylet may be inserted inside the endotracheal tube and used to facilitate intubation

   - The stylet is a plastic-coated metal wire that allows the endotracheal tube to be shaped to any desired configuration

   - *The tip of the stylet must be recessed $1/2$ inch from the end of the endotracheal tube to avoid trauma to the anatomical structures*

3. Connect the laryngoscope blade and handle

   a. Check the blade for a "white, bright, light"

   b. The curved (MacIntosh) blade is inserted into the vallecula. The soft tissue is then lifted and the glottic opening (the space between the vocal cords) visualized.

      - The term "vallecula" means "little valley" and is the space between the base of the tongue and the epiglottis

   c. The straight (Miller) blade is inserted under the epiglottis

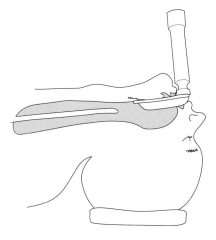

Figure 4-14   The straight blade is placed under the epiglottis.

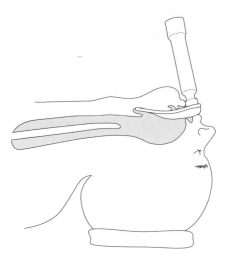

Figure 4-15   The curved blade is inserted into the vallecula.

4. Select and lubricate the appropriate size tube
   a. Females 7.5-8.0 internal diameter
   b. Males 8.0-8.5 internal diameter
   c. Best to have one half size smaller and one half size larger on hand
5. Attain proper head position
   a. Three axes must be aligned to achieve direct visualization of the larynx (mouth, pharynx and trachea)
   b. This is accomplished when the head is placed in the "sniffing" position - the head extended and neck flexed
      • If cervical spine injury is suspected, endotracheal intubation is performed with in-line stabilization of the head and neck

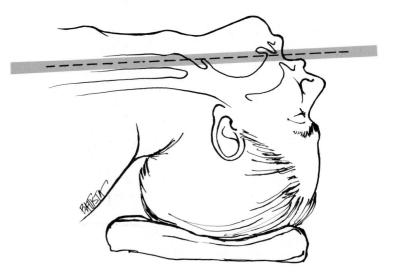

Figure 4-16   The "sniffing" position – the head is extended and the neck flexed.

6. Hyperventilate the patient with 100% oxygen

7. (Begin timing)**

   With the laryngoscope held in the LEFT hand

   - Insert the blade into the right side of the mouth, sweeping the tongue to the left
   - DO NOT USE THE TEETH AS A FULCRUM
   - Visualize the epiglottis, then the vocal cords
   - Insert the endotracheal tube from the right corner of the mouth through the vocal cords
   - Advance the endotracheal tube $1/2$ to 1" beyond the cords
   - Inflate the cuff (usually 6-10 ml of air) and ventilate the patient by attaching the bag-valve device to the endotracheal tube

   (End timing)

   **Time should not exceed 30 seconds*

Confirm endotracheal tube placement	Observe the rise and fall of the chest
	Perform a 5 point auscultation:
	• Auscultate breath sounds of the left and right lung fields at the apices and anterior bases
	• Auscultate over the epigastrium (should be silent)

Special
Considerations

1. Note the depth marking on the side of the endotracheal tube
    *   Usually between 19 and 23 cm in the average adult
2. After securing the ET tube, reassess depth markings
3. If breath sounds are absent bilaterally after intubation and gurgling is heard over the epigastrium, assume esophageal intubation
    *   Deflate the endotracheal tube cuff, remove the endotracheal tube and hyperventilate before reattempting intubation
4. If breath sounds are diminished on the left after intubation but present on the right, assume right mainstem bronchus intubation
    *   Deflate the endotracheal tube cuff, pull back the endotracheal tube slightly, reinflate the cuff and reevaluate breath sounds
5. Cricoid pressure (Sellick maneuver) may be applied to minimize gastric distention and aspiration and to aid placement of the endotracheal tube into the tracheal opening. Cricoid pressure should be maintained until the endotracheal tube cuff is inflated and the position of the tube is assured.
    *   The Sellick maneuver compresses and occludes the esophagus between the cricoid cartilage and the 5th and 6th cervical vertebrae

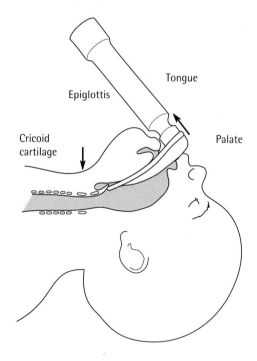

Figure 4-17   Application of cricoid pressure (Sellick maneuver).

Cautions

1. Should take no more than 30 seconds for procedure
2. Should be performed only by trained personnel

Complications
of Endotracheal
Intubation

1. Aspiration
2. Cuff leak
3. Laryngospasm
4. Bronchospasm
5. Inadvertent esophageal intubation
6. Inadvertent right mainstem bronchus intubation
7. Hypoxia due to prolonged or unsuccessful intubation
8. Dysrhythmias
9. Obstruction of the endotracheal tube
10. Trauma to the lips, teeth, tongue or soft tissues of the oropharynx
11. Increased intracranial pressure

TRANSTRACHEAL CATHETER VENTILATION

Description

Method of providing ventilation by insertion of a large-bore over-the-needle catheter into the cricothyroid membrane with intermittent jet ventilation

- Temporary procedure

Indications

Upper airway obstruction that cannot be relieved by other methods.

Obstruction may be due to:
- Edema of the glottis
- Fracture of the larynx
- Severe oropharyngeal hemorrhage

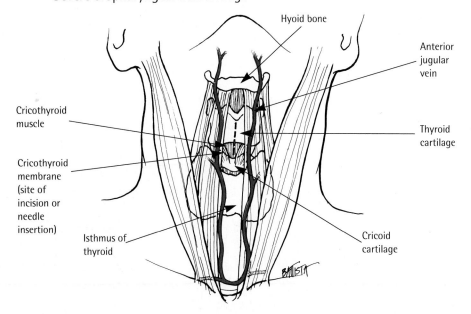

Figure 4-18   Anatomical landmarks for transtracheal jet insufflation and surgical cricothyroidotomy.

Procedure

1. Place patient in supine position and hyperextend the head and neck (if spinal injury suspected, maintain head and neck in neutral position)
2. Identify landmarks (thyroid cartilage, cricoid cartilage, cricothyroid membrane)
3. Cleanse site
4. Carefully puncture the skin in the midline directly over the cricothyroid membrane
5. Direct needle and syringe caudally at a 45° angle
6. Carefully insert needle and catheter through lower $1/2$ of the cricothyroid membrane, maintaining negative pressure as the needle is advanced
   - Aspiration of air signifies entry in the tracheal lumen
7. Advance the catheter over the needle until the catheter hub is flush with the skin
   - Hold the catheter hub in place to prevent displacement while removing the needle and syringe
8. Attach transtracheal ventilation system tubing to catheter
9. Observe rise and fall of the chest and auscultate for adequate ventilation
10. Secure catheter in place

Advantages

Allows rapid entrance to the airway for temporary ventilation and oxygenation

Disadvantages

1. Does not for direct suctioning of secretions
2. Does not allow for efficient elimination of carbon dioxide
3. Invasive procedure
4. Requires skilled rescuers to perform with frequent retraining

Complications

1. Asphyxia
2. Aspiration
3. Esophageal perforation if needle advanced too far
4. Hematoma
5. Thyroid perforation
6. Subcutaneous or mediastinal emphysema
7. Inadequate ventilation may lead to hypoxia and death

SURGICAL CRICOTHYROTOMY

Description

Creation of an opening into the cricothyroid membrane with a knife to allow rapid entrance to the airway for temporary ventilation and oxygenation

Indications	Upper airway obstruction that cannot be relieved by other methods

Obstruction may be due to:
- Edema of the glottis
- Fracture of the larynx
- Severe oropharyngeal hemorrhage

Procedure

1. Place patient in supine position
2. Identify landmarks (thyroid cartilage, cricoid cartilage, cricothyroid membrane)
3. Cleanse site
4. Stabilize thyroid cartilage and make a skin incision over the lower half of the cricothyroid membrane
5. Carefully incise through the cricothyroid membrane and listen/feel for air flow
6. With the scalpel in place, use a gloved finger (or forceps) to enlarge the hole horizontally
7. Insert an appropriately sized (average size 6.0-7.5) endotracheal tube into the cricothyroid membrane incision
8. Direct the endotracheal tube caudally into the trachea until the top edge of the endotracheal tube cuff disappears into the cricothyroid membrane incision
9. Inflate the endotracheal tube cuff and ventilate the patient with 100% oxygen
10. Observe rise and fall of the chest, assess bilateral breath sounds and auscultate the epigastrium
11. Secure the endotracheal tube to prevent dislodgement and note the centimeter marking on the endotracheal tube

Advantages

Allows rapid entrance to the airway for temporary ventilation and oxygenation

Disadvantages

1. Invasive procedure
2. Requires skilled rescuers to perform with frequent retraining

Complications

1. Asphyxia
2. Aspiration (blood)
3. Creation of a false passage into the tissues
4. Mediastinal emphysema
5. Hemorrhage or hematoma formation
6. Vocal cord paralysis
7. Hoarseness
8. Laceration of the trachea/esophagus

5 Adjuncts for Artificial Circulation

Objectives

Upon completion of this chapter, you will be able to:

1. Understand methods available for providing artificial circulation during cardiopulmonary arrest
2. Describe advantages and problems associated with mechanical chest compressors.
3. Describe the clinical indications for use of the pneumatic antishock garment (PASG).
4. List three indications for invasive (open-chest) CPR.

ALTERNATIVE CPR TECHNIQUES

IAC-CPR

Intermittent abdominal compression CPR

- Includes compression of the abdomen during the relaxation phase of chest compression
- Studies demonstrated improved survival for in-hospital resuscitation with this technique but not with out-of-hospital arrest

Simultaneous Ventilation, Abdominal Binding

1. Blood flow during external chest compressions results from an increase in intrathoracic pressure rather than direct pressure in an unknown percentage of humans in cardiac arrest
2. Simultaneous ventilation and abdominal binding techniques were devised to take advantage of the entire thorax as a pump during CPR
3. Studies have failed to demonstrate improvement in resuscitation success compared with standard CPR
4. Not currently recommended for treatment of patients in cardiac arrest

High-frequency CPR

1. Alternative CPR technique
2. Takes advantage of compression of the vascular structures during chest compression
3. High chest compression rates of 120/min yielded improved perfusion pressures and outcome in animals
4. More studies needed to determine efficacy for cardiac arrest victims

MECHANICAL CHEST COMPRESSORS

1. Not a substitute for manual external chest compression
2. Should be used as an adjunct by trained persons to optimize compression and reduce rescuer fatigue in prolonged resuscitative efforts
3. Should be used only in adults; efficacy and safety have not been demonstrated in infants and children
4. Can be manual or automatic

Advantages

1. Eliminate rescuer fatigue
2. Standardize the technique of CPR
3. Free trained persons to participate in the delivery of ACLS when there is a limited number of rescuers
4. Assure adequacy of compression when a patient requires continued resuscitation during transportation

Disadvantages

Potential for interrupting chest compressions for extended periods while setting up and starting the device

Cardiac Press

Characteristics

1. Hinged, *manually* operated device
2. Adjustable stroke
3. Applied with only brief interruption in manual CPR

Advantages

1. Modest cost
2. Ease of storage, transportation and assembly
3. Light weight
4. Minimal possibility of mechanical breakdown

Problems

1. Tendency for the compressor head to shift position
2. Slippage of stroke adjustment device so that the plunger does not compress the chest adequately

Automatic Chest Compressor (cardiac thumper)

Characteristics

1. Gas-powered plunger mounted on a backboard
2. Programmed to deliver AHA recommended CPR in a 5:1 compression to ventilation ratio that is 50% of the cycle length

Advantages

1. Does not require electrical power, powered by 100% oxygen gas
2. Compressions, ventilations can be adjusted as necessary
3. Eliminates variables such as operator technique and rescuer fatigue
4. Acceptable ECG can be recorded with compressor in operation
5. Patient can be defibrillated or transported without interrupting CPR
6. Hemodynamics produced are comparable to those produced during standard manual CPR

Problems

1. Sternal fracture
2. Expensive
3. Size
4. Weight
5. Restrictions on mobility

CPR VEST

Physiological Effects

Designed to take advantage of the thoracic pump mechanism of blood flow

Results

1. Demonstrated promise for improved hemodynamics during CPR
2. Clinical studies have focused on hemodynamics but have not assessed survival compared with standard CPR
3. *Experimental technique*; not recommended for routine use in cardiac arrest patients

PNEUMATIC ANTISHOCK GARMENT (PASG)

Physiological Effects

Provides circumferential pneumatic compression to the legs and abdomen producing a sudden increase in peripheral vascular resistance and mean arterial pressure

Clinical Indications   Hypovolemic shock secondary to bleeding in the lower half of the body

Routine use in cardiac arrest is not recommended since there is no documented evidence to indicate the PASG enhances survival of the cardiac arrest victim

INVASIVE (OPEN CHEST) CPR

General Principles
1. NOT an adjunct for maintaining artificial circulation
2. May provide near-normal perfusion of the brain and heart
3. Direct cardiac massage applied early in cardiac arrest after short period of ineffective closed-chest CPR can improve survival from cardiac arrest
4. Survival not improved when applied late (after more than 25 min total arrest time)
5. Necessitates well-coordinated team

Indications
1. Penetrating chest trauma
2. Consider in cardiac arrest caused by:
   - hypothermia
   - pulmonary embolism
   - pericardial tamponade
   - abdominal hemorrhage
3. Chest deformity where closed-chest CPR is not effective
4. Penetrating abdominal trauma with deterioration and cardiac arrest
5. Blunt trauma with cardiac arrest

EMERGENCY CARDIOPULMONARY BYPASS

General Principles
1. Studies have shown the feasibility of cardiopulmonary bypass in the treatment of selected patients in cardiac arrest
2. Bypass pump can be applied using the femoral artery and vein without requiring thoracotomy
3. Further studies needed to define the role of cardiopulmonary bypass in the management of patients in cardiac arrest

AIRWAY MANAGEMENT/ADJUNCTS FOR ARTIFICIAL CIRCULATION QUIZ

1. You have intubated a 60 year old female patient in cardiac arrest. Which of the following would indicate inadvertent esophageal intubation?

   a. subcutaneous emphysema
   b. external jugular vein distention
   c. gurgling sounds heard over the epigastrium
   d. breath sounds present on only one side of the chest

2. The average tidal volume that should be delivered when ventilating an adult with a bag-valve device is:

   a. 4-6 ml/kg
   b. 2-10 ml/kg
   c. 8-20 ml/kg
   d. 10-15 ml/kg

3. According to AHA guidelines, when ventilating a patient during a cardiac or respiratory arrest, the respiratory rate should be:

   a. 6-10 breaths/minute
   b. 8-15 breaths/minute
   c. 10-12 breaths/minute
   d. 15-30 breaths/minute

4. Which of the following flow rates may be used with a nasal cannula?

   a. 1-6 liters/minute
   b. 2-8 liters/minute
   c. 8-12 liters/minute
   d. 10-15 liters/minute

5. Which of the following statements regarding manually operated mechanical chest compressors is INCORRECT?

   a. these devices are expensive and difficult to store
   b. the compressor head of the device may shift position
   c. the stroke adjustment device may slip so that the plunger does not compress the chest adequately
   d. these devices may be used as an adjunct to optimize compression and reduce rescuer fatigue in prolonged resuscitative efforts

6. Use of the esophageal obturator airway (EOA) is considered a Class __ recommendation.

    a. Class I
    b. Class IIa
    c. Class IIb
    d. Class III

7. At the proper flow rate(s), which of the following percentages of oxygen may be delivered with a nasal cannula?

    a. 20-30%
    b. 25-45%
    c. 35-60%
    d. 60-80%

8. The most common cause of airway obstruction in the unresponsive patient is:

    a. the tongue
    b. the epiglottis
    c. foreign bodies
    d. teeth (dentures)

9. Successful placement of an endotracheal tube in an adult usually results in the depth marking on the side of the tube lying between the __ mark at the front teeth.

    a. 15 and 20 cm
    b. 19 and 23 cm
    c. 20 and 25 cm
    d. 16 and 22 cm

10. Select the INCORRECT statement regarding the use of an oropharyngeal airway.

    a. should be used only in conscious patients
    b. should be inserted only by persons properly trained in their use
    c. should be used when possible for unconscious patients who are not intubated
    d. incorrect insertion can displace the tongue into the hypopharynx and result in airway obstruction

11. The endotracheal tube size usually recommended for women is __ mm in internal diameter.

    a. 6.5-7.0
    b. 7.0-7.5
    c. 7.5-8.0
    d. 8.0-8.5

12. Your patient has a history of chronic emphysema and is complaining of chest pain radiating down his left arm. You have initiated oxygen therapy by nasal cannula at 2 liters/minute and note he continues to complain of pain and is becoming cyanotic.

    You should:

    a. have the patient rebreathe into a paper bag

    b. apply a simple face mask at 4 liters/minute

    c. reduce the amount of oxygen to 1 liter/minute via nasal cannula

    d. administer 100% oxygen via nonrebreather mask and be prepared to intubate and assist ventilations if necessary

13. Transtracheal jet insufflation is used to relieve life-threatening:

    a. cardiac tamponade

    b. pulmonary embolism

    c. tension pneumothorax

    d. upper airway obstruction

14. When tracheal suctioning is performed, suction is applied:

    a. only during insertion of the catheter

    b. only during withdrawal of the catheter

    c. during insertion and removal of the catheter

    d. it makes no difference when suction is applied

15. The bag-valve device:

    a. cannot be used in a spontaneously breathing patient

    b. is most effectively applied by a single, experienced rescuer

    c. should have a self-refilling bag that is easily cleaned and sterilized

    d. must have a pop-off valve to prevent generation of excessive pressure during ventilation of the cardiac arrest patient

16. Which statement concerning the automatic mechanical chest compressor is INCORRECT?

    a. this device is inexpensive and light weight

    b. this device delivers an optimal rate and depth of compression by eliminating operator fatigue

    c. defibrillation can be performed while the compressor is in operation

    d. if the compressor is improperly positioned or operated, ventilation or chest compression, or both, may be inadequate

17. Application of cricoid pressure will result in:

    a. closing of the oropharynx
    b. increasing the diameter of the airway
    c. closing of the esophagus to prevent aspiration
    d. lifting the tongue from the back of the oropharynx

18. The lower airway is BEST protected by:

    a. frequent suctioning
    b. an endotracheal tube
    c. an oropharyngeal airway
    d. an nasopharyngeal airway

19. The Venturi mask:

    a. is a specialized mask that provides a high gas flow with a fixed oxygen
       concentration
    b. is a hand-held device capable of delivering 100% oxygen that is used to assist or control
       ventilation
    c. is a specialized mask with a reservoir bag attached that, when connected to oxygen at 10-15
       liters/minute, provides nearly 100% oxygen
    d. is a specialized mask with an oxygen inlet valve that is highly recommended whenever mouth-to-
       mouth ventilation is needed

20. A soft, uncuffed rubber or plastic tube that is approximately 15-20 cm in length and usually well
    tolerated in conscious or semiconscious patients best describes the:

    a. suction catheter
    b. endotracheal tube
    c. oropharyngeal airway
    d. nasopharyngeal airway

21. Open chest CPR may be considered in all of the following situations EXCEPT:

    a. penetrating chest trauma
    b. cardiac arrest due to hypothermia
    c. penetrating abdominal trauma with deterioration and cardiac arrest
    d. routinely if conventional closed-chest CPR has not resulted in return of a spontaneous pulse after
       10 minutes

22. The name given the technique of applying cricoid pressure during endotracheal intubation is:

    a. Vagal maneuver
    b. Sellick maneuver
    c. Biot's maneuver
    d. Heimlich maneuver

23. The esophageal obturator airway (EOA):

    a. provides a route for endotracheal suctioning
    b. provides a route for medication administration
    c. requires visualization of the airway for insertion
    d. is frequently followed by immediate regurgitation when removed

24. A bag-valve device will deliver nearly 100% oxygen when it is supplied with:

    a. 4-6 liters of supplemental oxygen
    b. 6-10 liters of supplemental oxygen
    c. 10-12 liters of supplemental oxygen
    d. 10-15 liters of supplemental oxygen and a reservoir bag with O_2 supply tubing

25. Which of the following statements regarding the pneumatic antishock garment (PASG) is INCORRECT?

    a. is not recommended for routine use in cardiac arrest
    b. increases peripheral vascular resistance and mean arterial pressure by providing circumferential pressure to the legs and abdomen
    c. is recommended in the management of traumatic injuries to the thorax
    d. evidence does not indicate the PASG enhances survival of the cardiac arrest victim

26. Advantages of mechanical chest compressors include all of the following EXCEPT:

    a. eliminate rescuer fatigue
    b. interruption of chest compression for extended periods while setting up and starting the device
    c. free trained persons to participate in the delivery of ACLS when there is a limited number of rescuers
    d. assure adequacy of compression when a patient requires continued resuscitation during transportation

27. Ventilation should be interrupted for no more than _____ seconds during an intubation attempt.

    a. 10 seconds
    b. 30 seconds
    c. 45 seconds
    d. 60 seconds

28. The esophageal obturator airway (EOA) is contraindicated in:

    1. known esophageal disease
    2. patients who have ingested caustic substances
    3. children under the age of 16
    4. unconscious, apneic patients

    a. 1, 2
    b. 4
    c. 2, 3, 4
    d. 1, 2, 3

29. Select the correct statement regarding the simple face mask.

    a. provides definitive control of the airway
    b. the O_2 flow rate must be greater than 5 liters/minute to avoid accumulation of exhaled air in the mask reservoir
    c. preferred device for use in COPD patients because it provides precise O_2 concentrations
    d. can be used effectively to deliver high concentrations of oxygen in the apneic patient

30. When the oropharyngeal has been properly sized and placed, its proximal end should:

    a. rest comfortably on the patient's lips
    b. lie directly on the patient's front teeth
    c. lie directly behind the patient's front teeth
    d. protrude approximately $1/2$ inch from the patient's lips

31. The carina is:

    a. the opening between the vocal cords
    b. the space between the base of the tongue and the epiglottis
    c. a lid-like cartilaginous structure overhanging the entrance to the larynx
    d. the point where the trachea divides into the right and left mainstem bronchi

32. The maximum length of time for which a patient should be suctioned is:

    a. 5 seconds
    b. 10 seconds
    c. 30 seconds
    d. 60 seconds

AIRWAY MANAGEMENT/ADJUNCTS FOR ARTIFICIAL CIRCULATION QUIZ ANSWER SHEET

1. A　B　C　D

2. A　B　C　D

3. A　B　C　D

4. A　B　C　D

5. A　B　C　D

6. A　B　C　D

7. A　B　C　D

8. A　B　C　D

9. A　B　C　D

10. A　B　C　D

11. A　B　C　D

12. A　B　C　D

13. A　B　C　D

14. A　B　C　D

15. A　B　C　D

16. A　B　C　D

17. A　B　C　D

18. A　B　C　D

19. A　B　C　D

20. A　B　C　D

21. A　B　C　D

22. A　B　C　D

23. A　B　C　D

24. A　B　C　D

25. A　B　C　D

26. A　B　C　D

27. A　B　C　D

28. A　B　C　D

29. A　B　C　D

30. A　B　C　D

31. A　B　C　D

32. A　B　C　D

33. A　B　C　D

34. A　B　C　D

35. A　B　C　D

36. A　B　C　D

37. A　B　C　D

38. A　B　C　D

39. A　B　C　D

40. A　B　C　D

AIRWAY MANAGEMENT/ADJUNCTS FOR ARTIFICIAL CIRCULATION QUIZ ANSWERS

QUESTION	ANSWER	RATIONALE	JAMA PAGE REFERENCE
1	C	Absence of chest wall expansion and gurgling heard over the epigastrium indicate misplacement of the endotracheal tube into the esophagus.	2202
2	D	The adult patient should be ventilated with a tidal volume of 10-15 ml/kg.	2202
3	C	During cardiac or respiratory arrest, the AHA recommends the adult patient be ventilated at a rate of 10-12 breaths/minute (one breath every 5-6 seconds).	2202
4	A	The recommended flow rate for use with a nasal cannula is 1-6 liters/minute.	N/A
5	A	The manually operated mechanical chest compressor (cardiac press) is inexpensive, light weight and easy to store.	2204
6	C	The EOA is presently a Class IIb (POSSIBLY helpful) recommendation.	2202
7	B	1-6 liters/minute of oxygen delivered via a nasal cannula will deliver approximately 25-45% oxygen.	N/A
8	A	The most common cause of airway obstruction in the unresponsive patient is the tongue.	N/A
9	B	In the average adult, the endotracheal tube marking noted at the front teeth will be between 19 and 23 cm when the tube has been successfully placed.	2202
10	A	The oropharyngeal airway should be used only in UNCONSCIOUS patients. Use in the conscious patient may precipitate vomiting or laryngospasm.	2201
11	C	The recommended endotracheal tube size is 7.5-8.0 for women, 8.0-8.5 for men.	2201

12	D	This patient is showing signs of hypoxia. Administer 100% oxygen, be prepared to intubate and assist ventilations as necessary.	2199
13	D	Transtracheal jet insufflation is used to relieve life-threatening upper airway obstruction.	2203
14	B	Suction should be applied, using a rotating motion, only upon withdrawal of the catheter.	N/A
15	C	The bag-valve device may be used to assist ventilations in the spontaneously breathing patient; is most effectively applied using the two-rescuer technique; should have a self-refilling bag that is easily cleaned and sterilized; and should not have a pop-off valve.	2200
16	A	The automatic mechanical chest compressor (cardiac thumper) is heavy and expensive.	2204
17	C	Application of cricoid pressure (Sellick maneuver) results in compression of the esophagus, thereby reducing the risk of aspiration.	2201
18	B	The lower airway is best protected by an endotracheal tube.	2201
19	A	The Venturi mask provides a high gas flow with a fixed oxygen concentration. "B" describes an oxygen-powered mechanical breathing device. "C" describes a nonrebreather mask and "D" describes a pocket mask.	N/A
20	D	The nasopharyngeal airway is a soft, uncuffed rubber or plastic tube, approximately 15 cm in length, and usually well tolerated in conscious or semiconscious patients.	N/A
21	D	Open chest (invasive) CPR may be considered in penetrating chest trauma; cardiac arrest due to hypothermia, pulmonary embolism, pericardial tamponade, blunt trauma or abdominal hemorrhage; penetrating abdominal trauma with deterioration and cardiac arrest; and cases of chest deformity where closed-chest CPR is not effective.	2204

22	B	The Sellick maneuver is the name given to the cricoid pressure technique used during endotracheal intubation.	N/A
23	D	Removal of the EOA is frequently followed by immediate regurgitation. If the patient is unconscious, an endotracheal tube should be inserted and the cuff inflated before the EOA is removed. Suction must be readily available.	2202
24	D	A bag-valve device will deliver nearly 100% oxygen when supplied with 10-15 liters of supplemental oxygen and a reservoir bag.	N/A
25	C	The primary use for the pneumatic antishock garment (PASG) is for hypovolemic shock secondary to bleeding in the lower 1/2 of the body.	2204
26	B	"A disadvantage of any mechanical chest compression device is the potential for interrupting chest compressions for extended periods while setting up and starting them."	2204
27	B	Ventilation should be interrupted for no more than 30 seconds during an intubation attempt.	2201
28	D	The EOA is contraindicated in conscious patients, in children under 16, cases of known esophageal disease, for more than two hours and when caustic poisons have been ingested.	2202
29	B	When using the simple face mask, the O_2 flow rate must be than 5 liters/minute to avoid accumulation of exhaled air in the mask reservoir.	N/A
30	A	When the oropharyngeal has been properly sized and placed, its proximal end should rest comfortably on the patient's lips.	N/A
31	D	The carina is a projection of the lowest tracheal cartilage that forms a ridge between the openings of the right and left mainstem bronchi.	N/A
32	B	Suctioning should be applied for no more than 10 seconds.	N/A

33	A	When intubating with the curved laryngoscope blade, the tip of the blade is placed in the vallecula (the space between the base of the tongue and the epiglottis).	N/A
34	B	Endotracheal intubation should be preceded by some other form of ventilation. In the unconscious patient, insertion of an oropharyngeal airway and ventilation with a bag-valve device should be initiated to hyperventilate the patient prior to an intubation attempt.	2201
35	B	A simple oxygen face mask should deliver 40-60% oxygen at 8-10 liters/minute.	N/A
36	D	The oropharyngeal airway is inserted upside down into the mouth and rotated 180° when the distal tip reaches the soft palate.	N/A
37	A	The nasopharyngeal airway is a soft, *uncuffed* rubber or plastic tube — therefore there is no balloon that should be inflated with air.	N/A
38	D	The preferred technique for management of the airway in the unconscious patient without a gag reflex should include insertion of an oropharyngeal airway and ventilating with a bag-valve device until endotracheal intubation can be performed.	2201
39	A	ACLS medications which may be administered via the endotracheal tube include epinephrine, atropine and lidocaine. Naloxone may also be administered via this route.	2205
40	A	The highest possible concentration of oxygen (preferably 100%) should be administered as soon as possible to all patients with cardiac or pulmonary arrest or other patients with suspected hypoxemia, regardless of cause.	2205

Monitoring and Dysrhythmia Recognition 6

Upon completion of this chapter, you will be able to:

1. Describe the two types of myocardial cells and the function of each.
2. Describe the significance of each waveform in the cardiac cycle.
3. Describe the normal duration of the PR interval, QRS complex and QT interval.
4. Describe at least two methods of determining heart rate.
5. Name the primary and escape pacemakers of the heart and the inherent rates of each.
6. Define the absolute and relative refractory periods and their location in the cardiac cycle.
7. Describe correct electrode positioning for Leads I, II, III and MCL_1
8. Recognize the following dysrhythmias:
   - Sinus tachycardia
   - Sinus bradycardia
   - Premature atrial complexes
   - Paroxysmal supraventricular tachycardia (PSVT)
   - Atrial flutter
   - Atrial fibrillation
   - Junctional rhythms
   - AV blocks of all degrees
   - Premature ventricular complexes
   - Ventricular tachycardia
   - Torsades de Pointes
   - Ventricular fibrillation
   - Asystole

Definitions

1. Dysrhythmia = abnormal rhythm
2. Arrhythmia = absence of rhythm
   - Terms are used interchangeably

BASIC ELECTROPHYSIOLOGY

Myocardial Cell Types

1. Myocardial (working) cells (mechanical cells)
   - Contain contractile filaments that contract when the cells are electrically stimulated
2. Electrical cells (pacemaker cells)
   - Electrical conduction system cells form and conduct impulses very rapidly

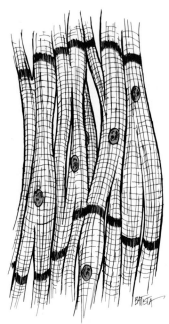

Kinds of Cardiac Cells	Where Found	Pimary Function	Primary Property
Myocardial cells	Myocardium	Contraction and relaxation	Contractility
Specialized cells of the electrical conduction system	Electrical conduction system	Generation and conduction of electrical impulses	Automaticity Conductivity

Figure 6-1   Cardiac cells. (Adapted with permission from Huszar, RJ: *Basic dysrhythmias: interpretation and management,* 2/e, St. Louis, 1994, Mosby-Year Book, Inc.)

Action Potential of a Myocardial Working Cell

1. Electrical impulses are the result of brief but rapid flow of positively charged ions (mainly Na+) back and forth across the cell membrane
2. The cardiac action potential is an illustration of the changes in the membrane potential of a cardiac cell during depolarization and repolarization

Phase 0 – Rapid Depolarization
- Also known as the "upstroke," "spike," or "overshoot"
- Begins when the cell receives an impulse
- Sodium moves rapidly into the cell through the fast sodium channels
- Potassium leaves the cell
- Calcium moves slowly into the cell through calcium channels
- Measures about +20 mV
- Cell depolarizes and cardiac contraction begins

Phase 1 – Early Repolarization

- Fast sodium channels close, stopping the rapid flow of sodium into the cell
- Potassium begins to reenter the cell and sodium begins to leave
- Measures about 0 mV (neutral, neither positively or negatively charged)
- Part of the absolute refractory period

Phase 2 – Plateau Phase (slow repolarization)

- Repolarization continues relatively slowly
- Calcium continues to enter the cell through slow calcium channels
- Part of the absolute refractory period

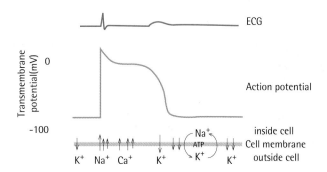

Figure 6-2   Action potential of the myocardial working cell.

Phase 3 – Final Rapid Repolarization

- The cell rapidly completes repolarization
- Calcium channels close
- Potassium rapidly flows out of the cell
- Active transport via the sodium-potassium pump begins restoring potassium to the inside of the cell and sodium to the outside of the cell
- The cell returns to its negative state due to the outflow of potassium
- The cell gradually becomes more sensitive to external stimuli until its original sensitivity has been restored (relative refractory period)

Phase 4 - Return to Resting State

- Corresponds with diastole
- Sodium and calcium remain outside the cell
- Potassium remains inside the cell
- The heart is "polarized" during this phase (ready for discharge)
- The cell will remain in this state until it's cell membrane is reactivated by another stimulus

THE ELECTROCARDIOGRAM

The P Wave

Represents atrial depolarization

The PR Interval

- Represents the length of time required for the atria to depolarize and the delay of the impulse through the AV junction
- Normally measures 0.12 to 0.20 second

The QRS Complex

- Represents ventricular depolarization (phase 0 of the action potential)
- Q wave = first negative deflection following the P wave
  - The normal Q wave is less than 25% of the amplitude of the R wave
  - The normal Q wave does not exceed 0.04 sec in duration
- R wave = first positive deflection after the P wave
- The QRS normally measures 0.04 to 0.10 sec in adults
- S wave = the negative deflection following the R wave

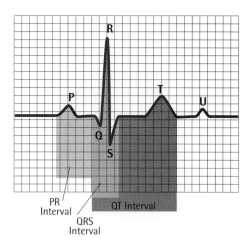

Figure 6-3   The electrocardiogram.

The ST Segment
- Represents early repolarization of the right and left ventricles
- Begins with the end of the QRS complex and ends with the onset of the T wave
- Is usually not depressed more than 0.5 mm in any lead

The T Wave
- Represents ventricular repolarization
- Is normally not greater than 5 mm in amplitude
- Peaked T waves are commonly seen in patients with hyperkalemia

The QT Interval
- Represents total ventricular activity (the time required for ventricular depolarization and repolarization to take place)
- Is measured from the beginning of the QRS complex to the end of the T wave
- Normally measures 0.36–0.44 sec but varies with the patient's heart rate (it is longer with slower heart rates and shorter with faster ones), age and sex
- A prolonged QT interval indicates a lengthened relative refractory period (vulnerable period) - which puts the ventricles at risk for life-threatening dysrhythmias (such as Torsades de Pointes) if a premature impulse occurs during this time period.

Determining Rate
Several methods may be used to calculate heart rate:

- Each one millimeter box (small square) represents 0.04 sec. There are 1500 boxes in one minute. To determine ventricular rate, count the number of small squares between two consecutive R waves and divide into 1500.
- Count the number of large squares (5 small boxes) between two R waves and divide into 300. This method is best used if the rhythm is regular, however, it may be used if the rhythm is irregular and a rate range (slowest and fastest rate) is given.
- Count the number of complete R waves within a period of 6 seconds and multiply that number by 10 to determine the rate for one minute.

ANALYZING A RHYTHM STRIP

Is the rhythm regular or irregular?

- To determine if the ventricular rhythm is regular or irregular, measure the distance between two consecutive R-R intervals (from a point on one R wave to the same point on the next R wave) and compare that distance with another R-R interval. If the ventricular rhythm is regular, the R-R intervals will measure the same.

- To determine if the atrial rhythm is regular or irregular, measure the distance between two consecutive P-P intervals (from a point on one P wave to the same point on the next P wave) and compare that distance with another P-P interval. If the atrial rhythm is regular, the P-P intervals will measure the same.

What is the atrial rate? What is the ventricular rate?

- To determine the ventricular rate, measure the distance between R-R.
- To determine the atrial rate, measure the distance between P-P.

Is the QRS complex wide or narrow?

- If the QRS measures .10 second or less (narrow), it is presumed to be supraventricular in origin.

- If it is greater than .12 second (wide), it is presumed to be ventricular in origin until proven otherwise.

- Do the QRS's occur uniformly throughout the strip?

Are P waves present?

- Are P waves present and uniform in appearance?
- Are P waves positive (upright) in Lead II?
- Is one P wave present before each QRS complex or are there more P waves than QRS complexes?
- Do the P waves occur regularly?

What is the duration of the PR interval?

- If the PR interval is less than 0.12 or more than 0.20 second, conduction followed an abnormal pathway or the impulse was delayed in the area of the AV node.

- Is the PR interval of conducted beats the same (constant) or does it vary?

DOMINANT AND ESCAPE PACEMAKERS OF THE HEART

Primary Pacemaker

1. Sino-Atrial (SA) node
2. Inherent rate = 60-100 beats/minute
3. Normally the pacemaker cells with the fastest rate control the heart at any given time
4. The SA node is normally the primary pacemaker of the heart because it possesses the highest level of automaticity

Escape Pacemakers

1. Atrio-Ventricular (AV) Junction
   - The AV *junction* is the AV node and the nonbranching portion of the bundle of His
     - The pacemaker cells in the AV junction are located near the non-branching portion of the bundle of His
   - If the SA node fails to generate an impulse at its normal rate, or stops functioning entirely, pacemaker cells in the AV junction will usually assume the role of pacemaker of the heart (but at a slower rate)
   - Inherent rate = 40-60 beats/minute

2. Ventricles
   - If the AV junction is unable to function, an escape pacemaker below the AV junction (the bundle branches and the Purkinje network) may take over at an even slower rate
   - Inherent rate = 20-40 beats/minute

ABSOLUTE AND RELATIVE REFRACTORY PERIODS

Definition

The time between the onset of depolarization and the end of repolarization results in periods during which cardiac cells may or may not be stimulated to depolarize. These are known as the *absolute* and *relative* refractory periods.

Absolute Refractory Period

1. Extends from the onset of the QRS to the peak of the T wave
2. Cardiac cells have not yet repolarized and cannot be stimulated to depolarize
3. Also known as the effective refractory period

Relative Refractory Period

1. Corresponds with the downslope of the T wave
2. Most of the cardiac cells have repolarized and can be stimulated to depolarize if the stimulus is strong enough
3. Also known as the vulnerable period

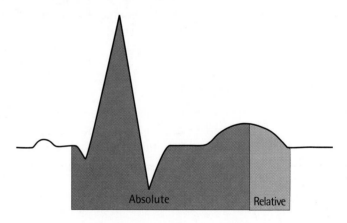

Figure 6-4　Absolute and relative refractory periods.

MECHANISMS OF IMPULSE FORMATION

Automaticity

1. The capability of cardiac cells to depolarize spontaneously without being stimulated by another source (such as a nerve)
2. Automaticity is normally present in the pacemaker cells of the SA node, the AV junction, and the ventricles

Reentry

1. An electrical impulse is delayed, blocked (or both) in one or more portions of the electrical conduction system while the impulse is conducted normally through the rest of the conduction system

2. This results in the delayed impulse entering cardiac cells which have just been depolarized by the normally conducted impulse and, if they have repolarized sufficiently, depolarizing them prematurely, producing ectopic beats and rhythms

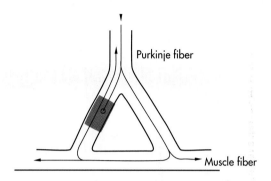

Figure 6-5   The mechanism of reentry.

CARDIAC CONDUCTION SYSTEM

Electrical Flow through the Heart

Originates in the SA node → AV node → bundle of His → left and right bundle branches → Purkinje fibers where the mechanical cells are stimulated

LOCATIONS FOR CHEST ELECTRODES

Lead I

- Positive electrode placed just below the left clavicle
- Negative electrode placed just below the right clavicle
- Provides information about the left lateral wall of the heart

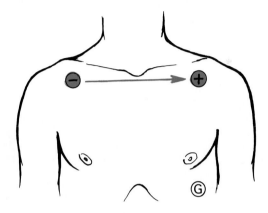

Figure 6-6   Lead I.

Lead II

- Positive electrode just below the left pectoral muscle
- Negative electrode just below the right clavicle
- Provides information about the inferior wall of the heart

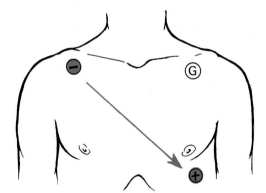

Figure 6-7   Lead II.

Lead III

- Positive electrode placed just below the left pectoral muscle
- Negative electrode placed just below the left clavicle
- Provides information about the inferior wall of the heart
- P waves seen in this lead are usually of lower amplitude than in leads I and II and are more likely to be biphasic (partly positive and partly negative)

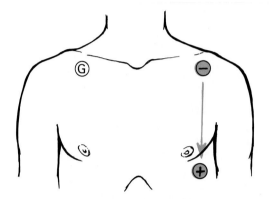

Figure 6-8   Lead III.

Lead MCL₁ (modified chest lead)

- Negative electrode placed just below the left clavicle
- Positive electrode placed to the right of the sternum at the fourth intercostal space
- Provides information about the anterior wall of the heart
- May prove useful in assessing the width of the QRS complex to differentiate supraventricular tachycardia (SVT) from ventricular tachycardia (VT)

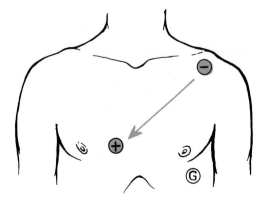

Figure 6-9   Lead MCL₁.

DYSRHYTHMIA RECOGNITION

Normal Sinus Rhythm
(NSR)

Rate:	60-100 beats/min
Rhythm:	Regular
P waves:	Uniform and upright in appearance
	One preceding each QRS complex
PRI:	.12-.20 sec
QRS:	< .10

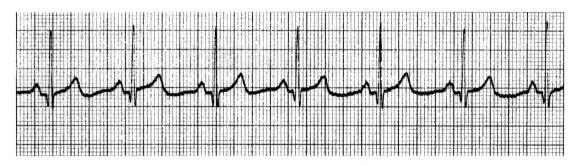

Figure 6-10   Normal sinus rhythm.

Sinus Bradycardia

Rate:	**< 60 beats/min**
Rhythm:	Regular
P waves:	Uniform and upright in appearance
	One preceding each QRS complex
PRI:	.12-.20 sec
QRS:	< .10

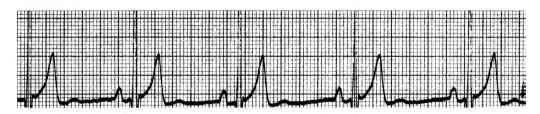

Figure 6-11   Sinus bradycardia.

Sinus Tachycardia

Rate:	**100-160 beats/min**
Rhythm:	Regular
P waves:	Uniform and upright in appearance
	One preceding each QRS complex
PRI:	.12-.20 sec
QRS:	< .10

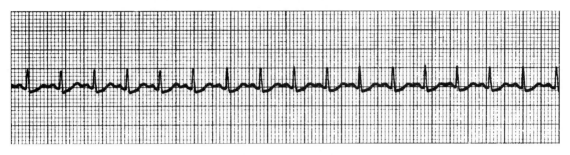

Figure 6-12   Sinus tachycardia.

Sinus Arrhythmia

Rate:	Usually 60-100 beats/min but may
	be faster or slower
Rhythm:	**IRREGULAR**
P waves:	Uniform and upright in appearance
	One preceding each QRS complex
PRI:	.12-.20 sec
QRS:	< .10

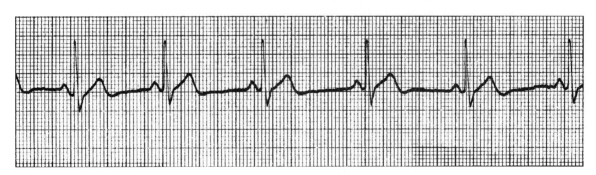

Figure 6-13   Sinus arrhythmia.

Premature Atrial
Complexes (PACs)

*Everything
normal & early*

Rate:	Usually normal, but depends on underlying rhythm
Rhythm:	Irregular due to PACs
P waves:	P wave of the early beat differs from sinus P waves
	Is premature
	May be flattened or notched
	May be lost in the preceding T wave
PRI:	Varies from .12–.20 when the pacemaker site is near the SA node, to .12 sec when the pacemaker site is nearer the AV node
QRS:	Usually < .10 but may be prolonged

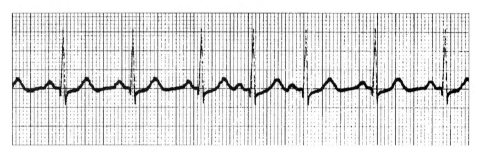

Figure 6-14   Premature atrial complexes (PACs).

Supraventricular
Tachycardia

Rate:	150–250/min
Rhythm:	Regular
P waves:	Atrial P waves differ from sinus P waves
	P waves are usually identifiable at the lower end of the rate range but seldom identifiable at rates >200
	May be lost in preceding T wave
PRI:	Usually not measurable because the P wave is difficult to distinguish from the preceding T wave; if measurable, is .12–.20
QRS:	< .10 sec

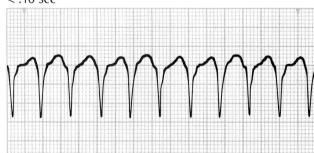

Figure 6-15   Supraventricular tachycardia (SVT). (Reproduced with permission from Huszar, RJ: *Basic dysrhythmias: interpretation and management* 2/e, St. Louis, 1994, Mosby-Year Book, Inc.)

Atrial Flutter

Rate: Atrial rate 250-350/min
Ventricular rate variable

Rhythm: Atrial rhythm regular
Ventricular rhythm usually regular
but may be irregular

P waves: **Saw-toothed, "flutter waves"**

PRI: Not measurable

QRS: Usually < .10 but may be widened if flutter waves are buried in
the QRS complex

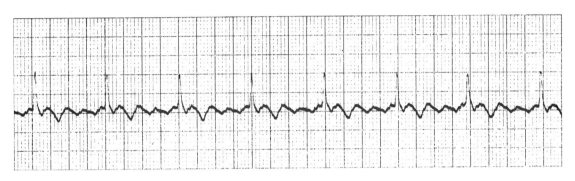

Figure 6-16   Atrial flutter.

Atrial Fibrillation

Rate: Atrial rate usually > 400
Ventricular rate variable

Rhythm: Atrial and ventricular very irregular
(regular, bradycardic ventricular
rhythm may occur as a result of
digitalis toxicity)

P waves: **No identifiable P waves**
Erratic, wavy baseline

PRI: None

QRS: Usually < .10

controlled rate <100
uncontrolled >100

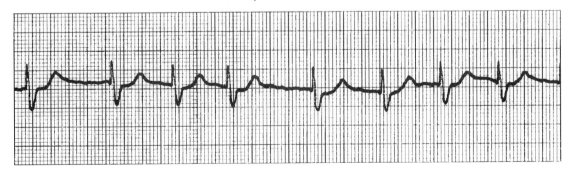

Figure 6-17   Atrial fibrillation.

Premature Junctional
Complexes (PJCs)

Rate: Atrial and ventricular rates dependent upon
           underlying rhythm

Rhythm: Irregular due to premature complex

P waves: **May occur before, during or after the QRS; if
seen, will be inverted (retrograde)**

PRI: If the P wave occurs before the QRs, the PRI will
usually be ≤ .12 sec

QRS: < .10

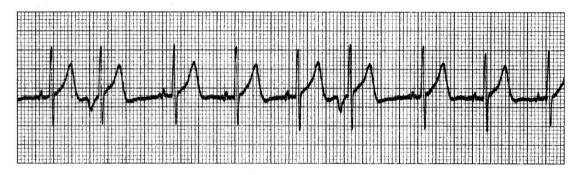

Figure 6-18   Premature junctional complexes (PJCs).

Junctional Rhythm

Rate: **40-60 beats/minute**

Rhythm: *Atrial and ventricular VERY REGULAR*

P waves May be occur before, during or after the QRS; if
seen, will be inverted (retrograde)

PRI: Not measurable unless the P wave precedes the
QRS; when present, will usually be ≤ .12

QRS: < .10

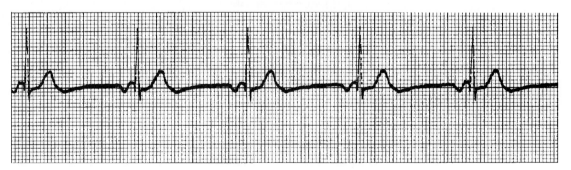

Figure 6-19   Junctional rhythm.

Accelerated
Junctional Rhythm

Rate: **60-100 beats/minute**
Rhythm: Atrial and ventricular VERY REGULAR
P waves: May be occur before, during or after the QRS; if
           seen, will be inverted (retrograde)
PRI: Not measurable unless the P wave precedes the
           QRS; when present, will usually be ≤ .12
QRS: < .10

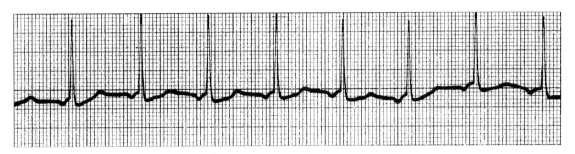

Figure 6-20   Accelerated junctional rhythm.

Junctional
Tachycardia

Rate: **100-180 beats/minute**
Rhythm: Atrial and ventricular VERY REGULAR
P waves: May be occur before, during or after the QRS; if
           seen, will be inverted (retrograde)
PRI: Not measurable unless the P wave
           precedes the QRS; when present,
           will usually be ≤ .12
QRS: < .10

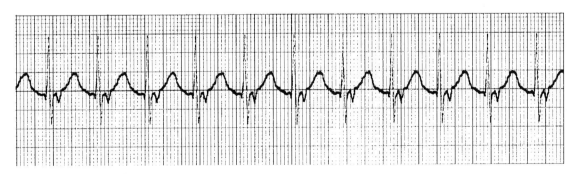

Figure 6-21   Junctional tachycardia.

Premature Ventricular Complexes (PVCs)

Bigeminy:
  PVC q other beat
Trigeminy:
  PVC q 3rd beat
Couplet:
  occur in pairs
Triplet:
  PVC's occur in 3's.

Rate: Atrial and ventricular rate dependent upon the underlying rhythm
Rhythm: Irregular due to PVC
           If the PVC is interpolated (sandwiched between two normal beats) the rhythm will be regular
P waves: There is no P wave associated with the PVC
PRI: None with the PVC because the ectopic originates in the ventricles
QRS: > .12
           Wide and bizarre
           T wave frequently in opposite direction of the QRS complex

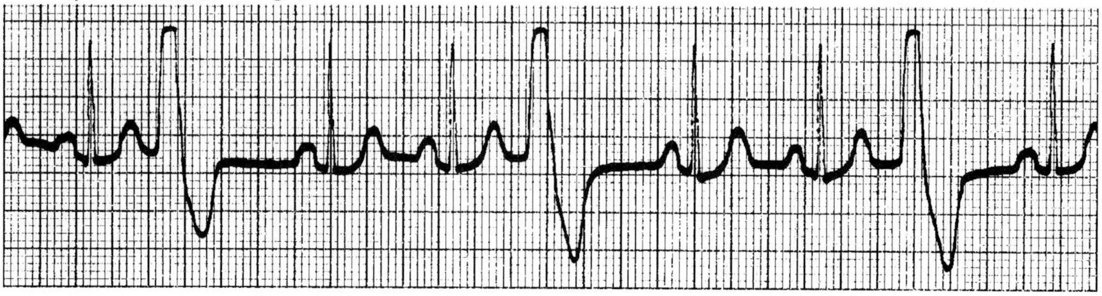

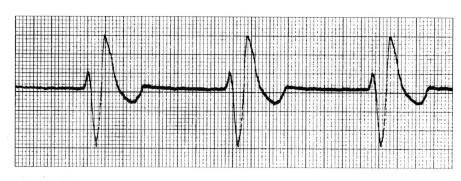

Figure 6-22   Premature ventricular complexes (PVCs).

Ventricular Escape Rhythm (Idioventricular Rhythm)(IVR)

Rate: Atrial not discernible; **ventricular 20-40 beats/minute**
Rhythm: Atrial not discernible, ventricular essentially regular
P waves: Absent
PRI: None
QRS: > .12

Figure 6-23   Idioventricular (ventricular escape) rhythm.

Accelerated	Rate:	Atrial not discernible; **ventricular 40-100 beats/minute**
Idioventricular Rhythm	Rhythm:	Atrial not discernible, ventricular essentially regular
(AIVR)	P waves:	Absent
	PRI:	None
	QRS:	> .12

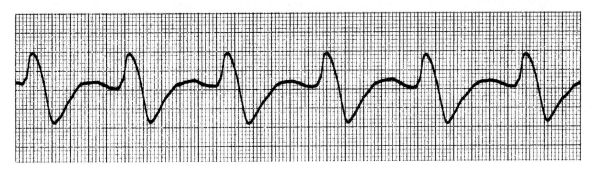

Figure 6-24   Accelerated idioventricular rhythm (AIVR).

Ventricular	Rate:	Atrial not discernible; **ventricular 100-250 beats/minute**
Tachycardia	Rhythm:	Atrial not discernible, ventricular essentially regular
(Monomorphic VT)	P waves:	May be present or absent; if present they have no set relationship to the QRS complexes - appearing between the QRS's at a rate different from that of the VT
	PRI:	None
	QRS:	> .12
		Often difficult to differentiate between the QRS and the T wave
	Note:	Three or more PVCs occurring sequentially are referred to as a "run" of VT.

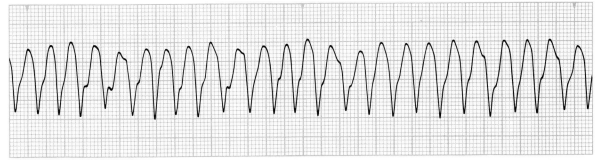

Figure 6-25   Ventricular tachycardia.

Torsades de Pointes   Rate: Atrial not discernible; **ventricular**
(TdP) (a type of   **150–250 beats/minute**
polymorphic VT)   Rhythm: Atrial not discernible, ventricular may be regular or irregular
                           PRI: None
                           QRS: > .12
                                      Gradual alteration in the amplitude and direction of the QRS

Torsades de Pointes (french for "twisting of the points") is a type of polymorphic VT associated with a prolonged QT interval. Symptoms associated with TdP are related to the ↓ cardiac output which occurs a result of the fast ventricular rate. Patients may complain of palpitations, lightheadedness, experience seizures or a syncopal episode. TdP is usually initiated by a PVC and may occasionally terminate spontaneously and recur after several seconds or minutes or it may deteriorate into VF.

The causes of long QT are many and include:[1]

1. Drug induced

   • Cyclic antidepressants (doxepin, imipramine, amitriptyline)

   • Phenothiazines (Haloperidol, Chlorpromazine, Thioridazine)

   • Type I antidysrhythmics (quinidine, procainamide, disopyramide, tocainide, mexiletine)

   • Organophosphate insecticides

2. Eating disorders (bulimia, anorexia)

3. Electrolyte abnormalities (hypomagnesemia, hypokalemia, hypocalcemia)

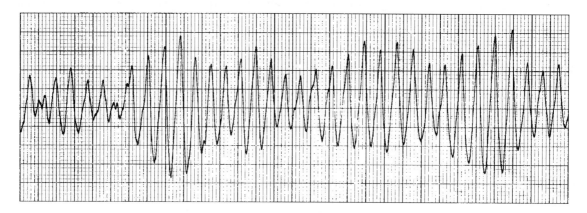

Figure 6-26   Torsades de Pointes.

Ventricular Fibrillation

Rate: Cannot be determined since there are no discernible waves or complexes to measure

Rhythm: Rapid and chaotic with no pattern or regularity

P waves: Not discernible

PRI: Not discernible

QRS: Not discernible

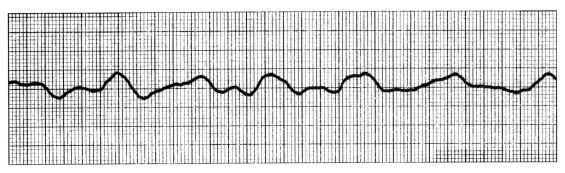

Figure 6-27   Ventricular fibrillation.

Asystole
(Ventricular Asystole,
Ventricular Standstill)

Rate: Ventricular usually indiscernible but may see some atrial activity

Rhythm: Atrial may be discernible, ventricular indiscernible

P waves: Usually not discernible

PRI: Not measurable

QRS: Absent

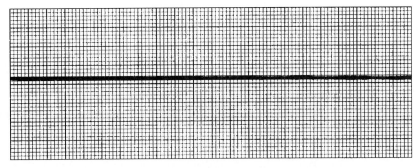

Figure 6-28   Asystole.

First Degree AV Block

Rate:	Atrial and ventricular within normal limits and the same
Rhythm:	Atrial and ventricular regular
P waves:	Normal in size and configuration
	One P wave for each QRS
PRI:	**Prolonged (>.20 sec) BUT CONSTANT**
QRS:	< .10

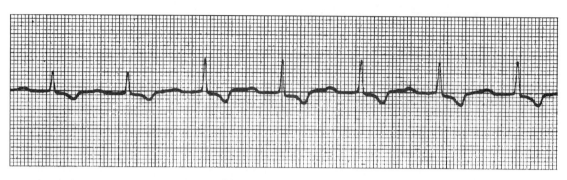

Figure 6-29   Sinus rhythm with first degree AV block.

Second Degree AV
Block, Type I
(Wenckebach,
Mobitz I)

Rate:	Atrial rate > ventricular rate, both are usually within normal limits
Rhythm:	**Atrial regular (P's plot through); Ventricular IRREGULAR**
P waves:	Normal in size and configuration
	Some P waves are not followed by a QRS (more P's than QRS's)
PRI:	**Lengthens with each cycle (although lengthening may be slight) until a P wave appears without a QRS**
QRS:	< .10 but is dropped periodically

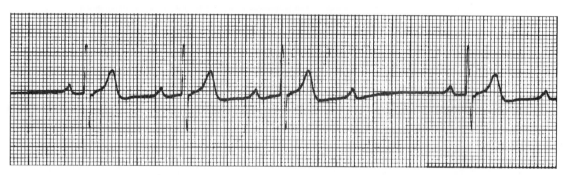

Figure 6-30   Second degree AV block, type I.

Second Degree AV Block, Type II (Mobitz II)	Rate:	Atrial rate > ventricular rate
	Rhythm:	**Atrial regular (P's plot through); Ventricular IRREGULAR**
	P waves:	Normal in size and configuration
		Some P waves are not followed by a QRS (more P's than QRS's)
	PRI:	May be within normal limits or prolonged but is CONSTANT FOR EACH CONDUCTED QRS
	QRS:	> .10 but is dropped periodically

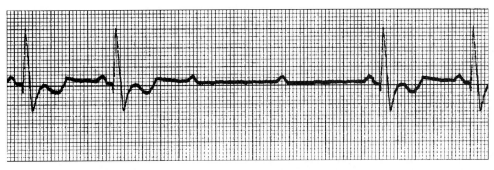

Figure 6-31   Second degree AV block, type II.

Second Degree AV
Block, 2:1 conduction

Rate:	Atrial rate > ventricular rate
Rhythm:	Atrial regular (P's plot through)
	Ventricular **REGULAR**
P waves:	Normal in size and configuration
	Every other P wave is followed by a QRS (more P's than QRS's)
PRI:	**CONSTANT**
QRS:	Within normal limits if the block occurs above the bundle of His (probably Type I)
	Wide if the block occurs at or below the bundle of His (probably Type II)
	Absent after every other P wave

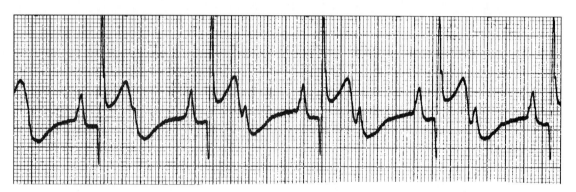

Figure 6-32   Second degree AV block, 2:1 conduction, probably Type I.

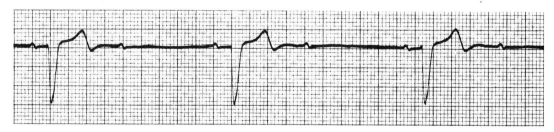

Figure 6-33   Second degree AV block, 2:1 conduction, probably type II. (Reproduced with permission from Conover, MB: *Understanding electrocardiography: arrhythmias and the 12-lead ECG* 6/e, St. Louis, 1992, Mosby-Year Book, Inc.)

Complete (Third
Degree) AV Block

Rate: Atrial rate > ventricular rate; ventricular rate determined by the origin of the escape rhythm

Rhythm: **Atrial regular (P's plot through); Ventricular REGULAR**

P waves: Normal in size and configuration
Some P waves are not followed by a QRS (more P's than QRS's)

PRI: **None** - the atria and ventricles beat independently of each other; no relationship between the P's and QRS's

QRS: Narrow or wide depending on the location of the escape pacemaker and the condition of the interventricular conduction system
Narrow → junctional pacemaker
Wide → ventricular pacemaker

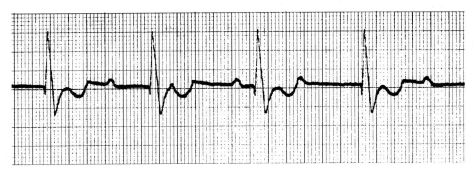

Figure 6-34   Complete (third-degree) AV block.

SINUS MECHANISMS – SUMMARY OF CHARACTERISTICS

TABLE 6–1.   SINUS MECHANISMS – SUMMARY

	RHYTHM	RATE	P WAVE	QRS	PRI	COMMENTS	CAUSES	SIGNS SYMPTOMS	TREATMENT
Sinus Rhythm	Regular	60–100	Upright	<.10	.12–.20				
Sinus Bradycardia	Regular	< 60	Upright	<.10	.12–.20		Normal in conditioned athletes. May be due to ↑ vagal tone (vomiting, straining at stool). May be seen after acute inferior wall MI or patient's on digitalis, beta-blockers, quinidine, verapamil.	May be asymptomatic. Fatigue, hypotension, syncope if ↓ cardiac output.	If symptomatic, ABCs, O₂, IV, atropine, pacer, dopamine, epinephrine, isoproterenol infusion.
Sinus Tachycardia	Regular	>100	Upright	<.10	.12–.20		Normal response to demand for O₂ due to fever, pain, anxiety, hypoxia, CHF, fright, stress, etc.	May be asymptomatic. Possible angina due to ↑ O₂ demand.	Treatment directed at correcting the underlying cause.
Sinus Arrhythmia	Irregular	Usually 60–100	Upright	<.10	.12–.20		Common in children and physically fit adults. Reflex vagal tone stimulation related to normal respiratory cycle.	Usually none.	

ATRIAL RHYTHMS – SUMMARY OF CHARACTERISTICS

TABLE 6-2. ATRIAL RHYTHMS – SUMMARY.

	RHYTHM	RATE	P WAVE	QRS	PRI	COMMENTS	CAUSES SYMPTOMS	SIGNS	TREATMENT
Supraventricular Tachycardia	Regular	160-250	Atrial P waves may be flattened or notched. P waves usually seen at lower end of rate range, seldom identifiable at rates > 200. May be lost in preceding T wave	<.10	May be <.12 if P wave seen.		In healthy persons, physical or psychological stress, hypoxia, excessive use of caffeine, etc. Usually occurs in patients with rheumatic heart disease, coronary artery disease (especially following acute MI), digitalis toxicity, respiratory failure or pre-excitation syndrome.	Sudden feeling of palpitations and severe anxiety. CHF, angina or shock may occur as a result of ↓ cardiac output and an ↑ need for oxygen if tachycardia persists.	Stable – ABCs, O₂, IV, vagal maneuvers, adenosine, verapamil. Unstable – ABCs, O2, IV, consider meds. If ineffective, administer sedation, synchronized countershock 50-100-200-300-360J.
Atrial Flutter	Regular or irregular	Atrial 250-350 Ventricular variable	Flutter waves "Sawtooth" "Picket-fence"	<.10	Not measurable	Significance of this rhythm depends on the ventricular rate. The more rapid the rate, the more serious the dysrhythmia.	Seldom occurs in the absence of organic heart disease. Seen in association with mitral or tricuspid valve disorders, digitalis toxicity, pericarditis, inferior wall MI.	May be asymptomatic. May sense palpitations. Signs of ↓ cardiac output if ventricular filling and coronary artery blood flow are compromised.	Depends on patient's presentation. Multiple options. If unstable with rapid ventricular rate, O₂, IV, consider meds, administer synchronized countershock 50-100-200-300-360J.

TABLE 6-2. CONTINUED   ATRIAL RHYTHMS – SUMMARY.

	RHYTHM	RATE	P WAVE	QRS	PRI	COMMENTS	CAUSES	SIGNS/SYMPTONS	TREATMENT
Atrial Fibrillation	Irregular	Atrial >400/min Ventricular = variable	None	<.10	Not measurable	Erratic, wavy, chaotic baseline. Inefficient movement of blood in the atria predisposes the patient to stroke.	Usually the result of some underlying heart disease and may occur intermittently or as a chronic rhythm. MI, COPD, coronary artery disease, CHF, cardiac valve disorders, rheumatic heart disease.	May be asymptomatic. May sense palpitations. Signs of ↓ cardiac output may be present and, if the patient has coronary artery disease, angina.	Depends on patient's presentation. Multiple options. If unstable with rapid ventricular rate, O_2, IV, administer sedation, synchronized countershock 100–200-300-360J.

JUNCTIONAL RHYTHMS – SUMMARY – SUMMARY OF CHARACTERISTICS

TABLE 6–3. JUNCTIONAL RHYTHMS – SUMMARY.

	RHYTHM	RATE	P WAVE	QRS	PRI	COMMENTS	CAUSES	SIGNS/SYMPTOMS	TREATMENT
Junctional Escape Rhythm	Regular	40–60	May occur before, during or after the QRS. If seen, is inverted.	<.10	If P wave is present, <.12		Digitalis toxicity Inferior wall MI Ischemia Hypoxia Valve surgery	May be asymptomatic. Signs of ↓ cardiac output if patient cannot tolerate ↓ rate or due to loss of atrial kick.	If symptomatic, ABCs, O₂, IV, atropine.
Accelerated Junctional Rhythm	Regular	60–100	May occur before, during or after the QRS. If seen, is inverted.	<.10	If P wave is present, <.12	This rhythm does not usually begin abruptly – it may first reveal itself with a few isolated PJCs	Usually due to excess digitalis. May also be due to inferior wall MI or post open heart surgery.	If the P wave is buried in the QRS, the patient will lose "atrial kick" which may produce sings of ↓ cardiac output.	Supportive care. Treat symptoms.
Junctional Tachycardia	Regular	100–180	May occur before, during or after the QRS. If seen, is inverted.	<.10	If P wave is present, <.12	If no P wave is seen and the rate is between 150 and 180, is often termed "SVT" because this rate range overlaps that of atrial tachycardia.	Usually due to excess digitalis. May also be due to inferior wall MI or post open heart surgery.	If the P wave is buried in the QRS, the patient will lose "atrial kick" which may produce signs of ↓ cardiac output.	Usually supportive care unless patient symptomatic. Treat symptoms.

VENTRICULAR RHYTHMS – SUMMARY OF CHARACTERISTICS

TABLE 6-4. VENTRICULAR RHYTHMS.

	RHYTHM	RATE	P WAVE	QRS	PRI	COMMENTS	CAUSES	SIGNS/SYMPTOMS	TREATMENT
Agonal Rhythm	Irregular	<20	Absent	>.12	Not measurable	Avoid giving lidocaine!	"Dying heart"	Signs/symptoms of ↓ cardiac output - severe hypotension, loss of consciousness, etc. May be pulseless although electrical activity seen on the monitor.	If pulseless, pulseless electrical activity. If pulse present, wide-QRS → pacing, support pressure with dopamine.
Idioventricular Rhythm (IVR)	Essentially regular	20–40	May be absent or, with retrograde conduction to the atria, may appear after the QRS (usually upright in the ST segment or T wave.)	>.12	Not measurable	Avoid giving lidocaine!	Myocardial infarction Digitalis toxicity	Severe hypotension possible, loss of consciousness or lightheadedness due to the profound bradycardia.	Wide QRS! If a pulse is present, pacing, support BP with dopamine if needed. If pulseless, PEA algorithm.
Accelerated idioventricular Rhythm (AIVR)	Essentially regular	40–100	May be absent or, with retrograde conduction to the atria, may appear after the QRS (usually upright in the ST segment or T wave)	>.12	Not measurable	Avoid giving lidocaine - this rhythm is PROTECTIVE! May be mistaken for VT if rate is not counted and the patient's condition assessed.	Myocardial infarction	Treatment necessary only if the patient shows signs/symptoms of ↓ cardiac output.	If rate 40–60 & patient is symptomatic, possible pacing/dopamine. If rate 60–100 and patient is hypotensive, dopamine may be ordered.
Monomorphic Ventricular Tachycardia	Usually Regular	>100	May be absent or, with retrograde conduction to the atria, may appear after the QRS (usually upright in the ST segment or T wave)	>.12	Not measurable	May result in ↓ cardiac output. May deteriorate to VF.	Often precipitated by R on T PVC. Myocardial irritability due to acute MI, coronary artery disease, CHF. May also be caused by toxicity from digitalis, quinidine, procainamide.	If conscious, patient may c/o palpitations, chest pain, shortness of breath. Signs and symptoms of ↓ cardiac output. Loss of consciousness, esp if VT is prolonged or sustained.	Stable = lidocaine 1–1.5 mg/kg, repeat with 1/2 dose q 5–10 min to max 3 mg/kg, hang drip. Unstable = synchronized countershock @ 100–200–300–360J. UNSYNC if there is a delay in synchronization or if the patient's condition is critical. Pulseless = CPR and defibrillation 200, 200–300, 360J
Polymorphic Ventricular Tachycardia (Torsades de Pointes)	Irregular	>150	Independent or none	>.12	Not measurable	Usually related to long QT interval	Drug induced (procainamide, quinidine, cyclic anti-depressants), electrolyte imbalance...	Palpitations, dizziness, syncope	If stable and time permits, electrical pacing is treatment of choice. Magnesium sulfate is drug of choice. If sustained, defib @ 200, 200–300, 360J
Ventricular Fibrillation	Chaotic	Not applicable	Absent	Absent	Absent	No cardiac output		Pulseless, apneic	CPR, defib 200, 200–300, 360J, resume CPR, intubate, IV, epi, defib 360 …
Asystole	None	Not applicable	None	None	None	No cardiac output	Acute respiratory failure, Extensive myocardial damage due to myocardial ischemia or rupture.	Pulseless, apneic	CPR, confirm rhythm in another lead, consider causes, consider pacing, epinephrine, atropine

AV BLOCKS – SUMMARY OF CHARACTERISTICS

TABLE 6-5. AV BLOCKS – SUMMARY

	RHYTHM	RATE	P WAVE	QRS	PRI	COMMENTS	CAUSES	SIGNS/SYMPTOMS	TREATMENT
First Degree AV Block	Regular	Usually 60–100	Upright	<.10	>.20 Constant	Conduction delay at the AV node	Drug therapy (quinidine, propranolol), inferior wall ischemia or infarction.	Usually asymptomatic	Supportive care Observe for increasing signs of block
Second Degree, Type I (Wenckebach, Mobitz I)	Irregular	Atrial > ventricular Both usually 60–100	Normal but some P waves are not followed by a QRS	<.10	Lengthens until a P wave appears without QRS	Almost always occurs at the level of the AV node and is usually a transient phenomenon	Inferior wall MI, drug therapy (digitalis, propranolol, verapamil), ↑ parasympathetic tone.	Usually asymptomatic. Possible hypotension and syncope if ventricular rate slow.	If symptomatic, ABCs, O₂, IV, atropine, pacer, possible dopamine.
Second Degree, Type II (Mobitz II)	Irregular	Atrial > ventricular	Normal but some P waves are not followed by a QRS	Usually >.10	May be normal or prolonged but is constant for each conducted QRS	This form of block usually occurs at or below the bundle of His May progress to complete block or asystole.	Anterior wall MI; severe coronary artery disease	May be asymptomatic. Possible angina due to increased O₂ demand.	If symptomatic, ABCs, O₂, IV, pacing, possible dopamine
Second Degree, 2:1 conduction	Regular	Atrial > ventricular	Two P waves for each QRS	May be <or> .10	Constant	Decision to term "Type I" or "Type II" is based on the patient's clinical condition and the width of the QRS I = QRS <.10 II = QRS >.10	See above	See above	Depends on width of QRS as outlined above
Complete (Third Degree) AV Block	Regular	Atrial > ventricular	More P's than QRS's	<.10 junction >.10 ventricles	None (No real PRI because the atria and ventricles beat independently of each other)	May result in ↓ cardiac output. May lead to asystole.	If block above the bundle of His = ↑ parasympathetic tone associated with inferior MI; from drugs (dig, Inderal) or from damage to AV node If block at or below the bundle of His = usually due to extensive anterior MI or extensive conduction system disease	Depends on the stability of the escape rhythm and patient response to ↓ rate.	If symptomatic and QRS narrow, ABCs O₂, IV, atropine, pacing, dopamine. If symptomatic and new wide-QRS, ABCs, O₂, IV, pacing, dopamine.

REFERENCES

1. Lefor N, Cardello F, Felicetta J, "Recognizing and Treating Torsades de Pointes," *Critical Care Nurse*, June 1992.

Electrical Therapy 7

Objectives

Upon completion of this chapter, you will be able to:

1. Define the terms unsynchronized and synchronized countershock.
2. Describe the differences in the delivery of energy relative to the cardiac cycle with unsynchronized and synchronized countershock.
3. Describe at least four factors affecting transthoracic resistance.
4. Describe proper placement of conventional defibrillator paddles.
5. Define and describe the procedure for performing a "quick-look".
6. Identify indications for delivery of unsynchronized countershock.
7. Identify indications for delivery of synchronized countershock.
8. Describe an automatic implantable cardioverter-defibrillator and management of the patient with this device.
9. Explain the precautions that should be taken when defibrillating a patient with a permanent pacemaker.
10. Describe the indications, precautions and technique for administering a precordial thump.
11. Explain the rationale for early defibrillation.
12. Explain the difference between the fully automated and semi-automated external defibrillator.
13. Describe at least three indications for emergent cardiac pacing.

Energy

1. The amount of current flowing through a circuit for any given voltage depends on the electrical resistance (**impedance**) of the circuit
2. If resistance increases, less current flows through the circuit
3. The amount of current penetrating the chest wall to shock the heart depends on the **transthoracic resistance** to the passage of that current
4. The strength (energy) of a countershock is expressed in **joules** (or watt-seconds)

Terminology

Countershock and cardioversion are GENERAL terms. Indicate specifically what TYPE of shock will be delivered:

- Unsynchronized countershock = defibrillation
  - The delivery of energy has no relationship to the cardiac cycle
- Synchronized countershock
  - Delivery of energy timed within milliseconds of the R wave in the cardiac cycle

FACTORS AFFECTING TRANSTHORACIC RESISTANCE (IMPEDANCE)

Delivered Energy

The higher the energy used for countershock, the lower the transthoracic resistance

Electrode (paddle) Size

To a point, transthoracic resistance decrease with increased paddle size

Paddle-Skin Coupling Material (Interface)

1. The skin acts as an electrical resistor between the paddles and the heart
2. If interface is not used:
   - skin surface burns
   - lack of penetration of current

Number and Time Interval of Previous Shocks

- The effect of the number of countershocks delivered on transthoracic resistance is cumulative
- Transthoracic resistance is also affected by the time interval between successive shocks
  - In the pulseless patient with VF or VT, three "stacked" shocks are delivered

Electrode (Paddle) Pressure

- Firm paddle pressure (approximately 25 pounds) may further decrease transthoracic resistance
- Exertion of firm pressure on the paddles may act to decrease transthoracic resistance by forcing exhalation

Phase of Patient's Ventilation

- Air is a poor conductor of electricity
- Transthoracic resistance appears to be lowest when countershock is performed during the expiratory phase of respiration because the distance between the paddles and the heart is decreased

Interelectrode (Paddle) Distance

- The recommended position for paddle placement is placement of one paddle to the right of the upper sternum just below the clavicle and the other just to the left of the nipple in the **midaxillary** line
- Anterior-posterior paddle positioning may also be used. One paddle is placed to the left of the lower sternal border and the other is positioned behind the heart.
- Insufficient data to indicate that one position is superior to the other

QUICK-LOOK PADDLES

Procedure

- Apply gel to defibrillator paddles or defibrillator pads to the patient's chest
- Turn the lead selector on the monitor/defibrillator to "paddles"
- Apply the paddles to the patient's chest
  - The paddles will function as electrodes, monitoring the patient's cardiac rhythm
- Precaution: removal of the paddles from the patient's chest while in "paddle" mode will result in artifact display on the cardiac monitor. The paddles must remain in contact with the patient's chest to monitor the patient's cardiac rhythm

DEFIBRILLATION – PROCEDURE

Purpose

1. Defibrillation does not "jump start" the heart
2. The purpose of defibrillation is to produce momentary asystole
   - The shock attempts to completely depolarize the myocardium and provide an opportunity for the natural pacemaker centers of the heart to resume normal activity
3. With unsynchronized shocks (defibrillation), the capacitors discharge when the shock controls (discharge buttons) are depressed
   - Unsynchronized shocks have no relation to the cardiac cycle
4. Electric shocks produce parasympathetic discharge
   - Routine shocking of asystole is strongly discouraged
   - Shocking asystole could eliminate any possibility for return of spontaneous cardiac activity

Operating the Defibrillator

1. Locate on/off switches
2. Patient leads
3. Quick look
   - Paddles used as electrodes
4. Determine mode appropriate for patient rhythm and condition
   - Synchronized mode
   - Unsynchronized mode = defibrillation
5. Locate charge button
   - On paddles
   - On machine
6. Discharge buttons
7. Hands-free defibrillation

Procedure for
Defibrillation

1. Apply conductive material to the paddles (gel) or chest wall (defib pads)
   - Remove nitroglycerin paste, patches, etc. from patient's chest if present
     - The aluminized backing used on some transdermal delivery systems can lead to electric arcing during defibrillation with explosive noises, smoke, visible arcing, patient burns and impaired transmission of current[1]
2. Turn on defibrillator
3. Select appropriate energy level for clinical situation
4. Place paddles on the chest and apply firm pressure
5. Charge paddles
6. State and LOOK to be sure area is clear
   a. Look all around (360°)
   b. "All clear!"
7. Press both discharge buttons simultaneously to deliver shock

DEFIBRILLATION - INDICATIONS

Ventricular
Fibrillation,
Pulseless
Ventricular
Tachycardia

Assess ABCs

CPR until defibrillator available

Precordial thump (if witnessed)

Defibrillate with 200J, 200-300J, 360J

- Leave the paddles in place on the chest between shocks (or use adhesive defibrillation pads for remote defibrillation)
- Visually reconfirm rhythm between defibrillations

Continue CPR

Intubate at once (confirm tube placement)

IV access

- Large-bore IV
- Antecubital or external jugular vein if no IV in place at time of arrest
- Normal saline or lactated Ringer's solution

Epinephrine 1 mg IV q 3-5 min

- If IV access delayed, endotracheal (ET) dose is 2-2.5 mg diluted in 10 ml of normal saline or distilled water
- If administered IV, follow with 20 ml bolus of IV fluid and elevate extremity

Defibrillate with 360J within 30-60 sec

REFRACTORY VF

Lidocaine 1-1.5 mg/kg IV push (may repeat with same dose every 5-10 min for maximum dose of 3 mg/kg)

Defibrillate with 360J within 30-60 seconds

Epinephrine 1 mg IV (or appropriate alternative)

Defibrillate with 360J within 30-60 seconds

Bretylium 5 mg/kg IV bolus

Pattern should be drug-shock, drug-shock

If the patient converts and refibrillates, use the same energy as the last successful shock

Unstable VT
(monomorphic)
with a Pulse

Energy delivery in unstable VT is usually synchronized @ 100, 200, 300, and 360J, however, *if there is an undue delay in synchronization, or if clinical conditions are critical, UNSYNC (defibrillate) at same energy.*

| Management of Polymorphic VT (Torsades de Pointes is a type of polymorphic VT) | 1. Treatment of choice is transcutaneous (overdrive) pacing
2. Drug of choice is magnesium sulfate 1-2 g IV over 1-2 minutes followed by same amount infused over 1 hour
3. Isoproterenol 2-10 μg/min may be considered |

Assess ABCs

Administer oxygen

Establish IV access

Administer sedation whenever possible

Unsynchronized countershock @ 200, 200-300, 360J

SYNCHRONIZED COUNTERSHOCK (CARDIOVERSION)

| Purpose | 1. Synchronized countershock reduces the potential for delivery of energy during the vulnerable period of the T wave (relative refractory period)
2. A synchronizing circuit allows the delivery of a countershock to be "programmed"
   • Searches for the peak of the QRS complex (R wave deflection)
   • Delivers the shock a few milliseconds after the highest part of the R wave |
| Procedure for Synchronized Countershock | 1. If awake and time permits, administer sedation
2. Apply conductive material to the paddles (gel) or chest wall (defib pads)
   • Remove nitroglycerin paste, patches, etc. from patient's chest if present
3. Turn on defibrillator
4. Select appropriate energy level for clinical situation
5. Press synchronizer switch/button
6. Assure machine sensing of R wave
7. Place paddles on the chest and apply firm pressure
8. Charge paddles
9. State and LOOK to be sure area is clear
   a. Look all around (360⁻)
   b. "All clear!"
10. Press both discharge buttons simultaneously to deliver shock |

	SYNCHRONIZED COUNTERSHOCK - INDICATIONS

Unstable VT with a Pulse

1. Signs/symptoms:
   - Dyspnea
   - Chest pain
   - Ischemia
   - Infarction
   - Hypotension
   - Pulmonary edema, congestive heart failure
   - Decreased level of consciousness
2. Precordial thump *only* if defibrillator and pacemaker immediately available
3. Consider medications
   - If the patient displays serious signs and symptoms, prepare for immediate countershock
4. Administer sedation whenever possible
5. Synchronized countershock
   - 100J, 200J, 300J, 360J

NOTE: If undue delay in synchronization, or if clinical conditions are critical, UNSYNC (defibrillate) at same energy.

Unstable PSVT

1. Unstable
   - Dyspnea
   - Ischemia
   - Infarction
   - Chest pain
   - Congestive heart failure/pulmonary edema
   - Unconscious
   - Hypotension
2. Management of the unstable patient in PSVT
   - Administer oxygen
   - Establish IV access
   - Consider medications
   - Administer sedation whenever possible
   - Synchronized countershock
     - 50, 100, 200, 300, 360J

Atrial Fibrillation - with a RAPID ventricular response, unstable patient

Synchronized countershock with 100, 200, 300, 360J

Atrial Flutter with a RAPID ventricular response - unstable patient

Synchronized countershock with 50, 100, 200, 300, 360J

Complications	If ventricular fibrillation occurs during the course of synchronization:

- Check pulse, check rhythm
- Turn off the synchronizer switch
- Defibrillate

AUTOMATIC IMPLANTABLE CARDIOVERTER–DEFIBRILLATOR (AICD)

Indications	Indicated for treatment of patients suffering from or at risk for sudden cardiac arrest

- Candidates for an AICD will have survived at least one episode of cardiac arrest due to either VT or VF, not associated with an acute MI OR
- Have recurrent VT that does not respond to conventional antidysrhythmic drug therapy

Patient Identification	1. Patients are asked to wear a medic alert tag and carry a unit identification card
	2. The I.D. card indicates:

- Type of unit
- Date of implantation
- Rate parameter (if any is used)
- If PDF (probable density function) is ON (being used as a determinant for shocks) or OFF (not being used)

The AICD	1. Delivers a shock of approximately 25-30 joules[2]
	2. Functions using two separate ventricular patches and two separate pacemaker leads that sense cardiac events
	3. Two pacing leads are placed on the epicardium and connected to the AICD

- Two patches are either sewn to the epicardium or placed outside the pericardial sac
- The leads from the pacing electrodes are tunneled under the ribs and connected to the device's generator, which is placed in the left upper quadrant of the abdomen

4. Each device is individually programmed so that when the monitored ventricular rate exceeds that of the preprogrammed rate, the device delivers a shock through the patches to restore a sinus rhythm

- The device requires 10-35 seconds to sense VT or VF and to charge it's capacitors prior to the delivery of a shock

- Once a shock is delivered, the device senses the rhythm. If a sinus rhythm has not been restored, the AICD will discharge again. This sequence can be repeated so that up to three (some models are programmed to deliver 4-6) shocks are delivered within a 2 minute period.

- If, at the end of the last shock, sinus rhythm has not been restored, the device will not fire again unless sinus rhythm resumes for a period of at least 35 seconds.

- If sinus rhythm is successfully restored and maintained for at least 35 seconds, the device can recycle and deliver a series of additional shocks if VT or VF recur[3]

- AICDs now available have the ability to perform overdrive pacing in addition to synchronized countershock, and defibrillation.

Managing the Patient with an AICD

1. Treatment of the patient with an AICD is no different that treatment of patients without them

2. Care should be taken to ensure that paddles or defib pads are not placed directly over the AICD present in the left upper quadrant of the abdomen

- Direct defibrillation discharges applied to the AICD can permanently damage its circuitry

3. Though the rescuer may feel the shock and experience pain, it is not dangerous

- Studies have shown that approximately 2 joules of energy are delivered at the body surface when the AICD discharges internally

- Although the energy is enough to be felt by the rescuer and may cause a momentary tingling sensation, it is not enough to cause physiologic harm

4. ECG monitoring devices will function normally and are not adversely affected by these discharges

| AICD Malfunction | Malfunction is uncommon but significant |
| | Most devices discharge when the rate becomes faster than the pre-programmed rate specific to each device |

- If the heart rate becomes > 170 beats/min, the device may discharge
- May occur with rapid atrial fibrillation or PSVT
- Patient may exhibit symptoms but may not lose consciousness

PERMANENT PACEMAKERS

| Precautions | Defibrillator paddles or self-adhesive electrodes should be placed at least 5 inches from the pulse generator of permanent pacemakers since it is possible for defibrillation to cause pacemaker malfunction. |

PRECORDIAL THUMP

| Indications | Class IIb (Possibly helpful) |

1. Ventricular Fibrillation
   - Use of the precordial thump should never be allowed to delay defibrillation
   - *Witnessed* arrest if a defibrillator is not immediately available
2. Ventricular Tachycardia
   - Never initiate in a patient in VT with a pulse unless a defibrillator and pacemaker are immediately available
   - May cause VT to deteriorate to VF, asystole or pulseless electrical activity

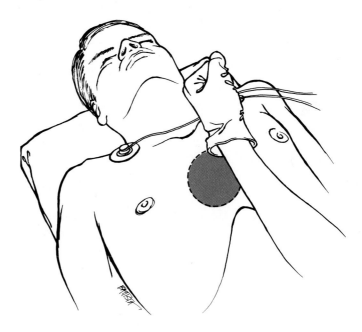

Figure 7-1   The precordial thump.

Contraindications	• Infants and children
	• Is an ACLS technique - *should not be taught to lay rescuers*

Method	1. Raised fist 8-10 inches above the chest (no more than 12 inches)
	2. *Single* thump delivered to the center of the sternum
	3. Recheck pulse and rhythm

AUTOMATED EXTERNAL DEFIBRILLATION (AED)

Principle of Early Defibrillation	"All BLS personnel must be trained to operate, equipped with, and permitted to operate a defibrillator if in their professional activities they are expected to respond to people in cardiac arrest."[4]

Rationale for Early Defibrillation	1. The most frequent rhythm seen in sudden cardiac arrest is VF.
	2. The most effective treatment for VF is electrical defibrillation.
	3. The probability of successful defibrillation diminishes rapidly over time.
	4. VF tends to convert to asystole within a few minutes.

What is an AED?	AED (automated external defibrillator)
	• An external defibrillator with a cardiac rhythm analysis system
	• Senses and records the rhythm, and if indicated, delivers an electrical shock
	• Shock is delivered by means of two adhesive pads applied to the patient (upper-right sternal border, lower-left ribs over the cardiac apex)
	• The adhesive pads have two functions:
	• Record the rhythm
	• Deliver the shock

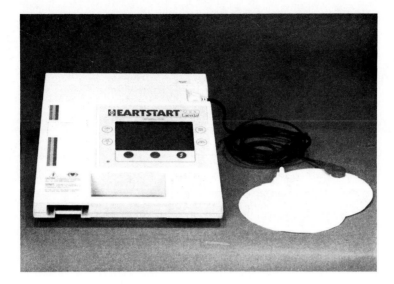

Figure 7-2   The Laerdel Heartstart 3000. (Reproduced with permission from Huszar, RJ: *Early defibrillation*, St. Louis, 1991, Mosby-Year Book, Inc.)

Types of
Automated
External
Defibrillators
(AEDs)

Fully automated defibrillator

- Requires that the defib pads be attached to the patient and the machine turned on
- Machine analyzes the rhythm. If VF (or VT above a preset rate) is present, machine charges its capacitors and delivers a shock

Semi-automated (shock-advisory) devices

- Requires operator to press an "analyze" control to initiate rhythm analysis and press a "shock" control to deliver the shock
- Shock control is pressed only when the device identifies VF (or VT above a preset rate) and "advises" the operator to press the shock control
- Never enters the analysis mode unless activated by the operator
- Leaves final decision of whether to shock to the operator

Automated
Analysis of Cardiac
Rhythms

1. Microprocessor analyzes multiple features of the surface ECG signal
   - Frequency
   - Amplitude
   - Integration of frequency and amplitude (such as slope or wave morphology)
2. Safety "filters" check for false signals:
   - Radio transmissions
   - Poor electrode contact
   - 60-cycle interference
   - Loose electrodes
3. AEDs take multiple "looks" at the patient's rhythm - each lasting a few seconds
   - If several "looks" confirm the presence of a rhythm for which a shock is indicated and other checks are consistent with a nonperfusing cardiac status:
     - Fully automated defibrillator will charge and deliver a shock
     - Semi-automated device will signal (written message, visual alarm or voice-synthesized statement) the operator that a shock is advised

AED Guidelines

1. AEDs should not be put in analysis mode until all movement, particularly the movement of patient transport, has ceased.
2. The AHA recommends the AED be attached only to those patients who are pulseless and apneic.
3. ACLS providers should NOT remove the AED and attach a separate conventional defibrillator unless the AED does not have a rhythm display screen
4. If a patient remains in VF after the delivery of three stacked shocks by the AED, ACLS personnel should enter the ACLS VF sequence at that point - i.e., continue CPR, intubate at once, establish IV access, administer epinephrine, etc.

Interruption of CPR

1. The patient should not be touched while the AED analyzes the rhythm, charges its capacitors and delivers the shocks
2. Chest compressions and ventilations must cease while the device is operating
3. The time between activating the rhythm analysis system (which is when CPR must stop) and the delivery of a shock averages 10-15 seconds

Advantages of Automated External Defibrillators	1. Less training required to operate and maintain skills
	2. Speed of operation (delivery of first shock) faster than that with conventional defibrillators
	3. Permits remote, "hands-free" defibrillation

| Disadvantages of AEDs | 1. Liquid crystal display that may be less suitable than the displays of conventional defibrillators |
| | 2. Lowest energy setting for the AED is 200J - high for patients weighing less than 50 kg |

Age and Weight Guidelines

Attach AEDs only to patients in cardiac arrest who weigh more than 90 pounds

- AEDs have a minimum energy level of 200J which is high for patients weighing less than 50 kg (110 pounds)

TRANSCUTANEOUS CARDIAC PACING

Advantages

- Ease of application
- Lack of significant pain
- Safety
- Least invasive pacing technique available
- Can be used effectively by prehospital personnel, nurses and other non-physician providers with appropriate training

Special Considerations

1. Failure to capture may be related to electrode placement or patient size
2. Patients with barrel-shaped chests and large amounts of intrathoracic air conduct electricity poorly and may be refractory to capture
3. A large pericardial effusion or tamponade will increase the output required for capture
4. If defibrillation is necessary when pacing electrodes have been applied to the chest, the defib pads and paddles should be placed 2-3 cm from the pacer electrodes to prevent arcing

Emergency Pacing -
Indications

1. Hemodynamically compromising (BP < 80 systolic, change in mental status, myocardial ischemia, pulmonary edema) bradycardias

   - Complete heart block
   - Symptomatic second degree heart block
   - Symptomatic sick sinus syndrome
   - Drug-induced bradycardias (digoxin, β- blockers, calcium channel blockers, procainamide)
   - Permanent pacemaker failure
   - Idioventricular rhythms
   - Symptomatic atrial fibrillation with a slow ventricular response
   - Refractory bradycardia during resuscitation of hypovolemic shock

2. Bradycardia with malignant escape rhythms unresponsive to pharmacologic therapy

3. Overdrive pacing of refractory tachycardia

   - Supraventricular or ventricular (in special situations refractory to pharmacologic therapy or countershock)

4. Bradysystolic cardiac arrest

   - Not routinely recommended
   - If used at all, should be used as early as possible after onset of arrest

TRANSVENOUS PACING

Procedure

Endocardial stimulation of the patient's right ventricle by means of an electrode introduced into a central vein

Placement of the catheter tip into the apex of the right ventricle is the key to success

Transcutaneous pacing can be used to temporarily stabilize the patient until a transvenous pacemaker can be inserted

TABLE 7-1. ELECTRICAL THERAPY - SUMMARY.		
Synchronized Countershock	PSVT	50-100-200-300-360J
	Atrial Flutter	50-100-200-300-360J
	Atrial Fibrillation	100-200-300-360J
	VT	100-200-300-360J
Unsynchronized Countershock	VT (delay in synchronization or critically unstable)	100-200-300-360J
	Polymorphic VT (unstable - sustained rhythm)	200, 200-300, 360J
	VF	200, 200-300, 360J

REFERENCES

1. Panacek EA, Munger MA, Rutherford WF, Gardner SF. Report of nitropatch explosions complicating defibrillation. *Am J Emerg Med.* 10:128-129, 1992.

2. Ziga R. Keeping pace. *Emergency.* February 1991.

3. Iverson WR, Harmann JR, Foy BK, Stamato, NJ. AICDs spark hope for cardiac care. *JEMS,* September 1989.

4. American Heart Association: *Automated External Defibrillation, Textbook of advanced cardiac life support,* Dallas, American Heart Association, 1990.

MONITORING & DYSRHYTHMIA RECOGNITION/ ELECTRICAL THERAPY QUIZ

1. The adhesive pads used with the automated external defibrillator should be placed:

   a. anterior chest, posterior thorax

   b. below the left clavicle nd at the cardiac apex

   c. below the right nipple and below the left nipple

   d. upper-right sternal border and lower-left ribs over the cardiac apex

2. In sinus arrhythmia, a gradual increasing of the heart rate is usually associated with:

   a. expiration

   b. inspiration

   c. excessive caffeine intake

   d. early signs of congestive heart failure

3. You have delivered a synchronized countershock with 50J to an unstable patient with paroxysmal supraventricular tachycardia (PSVT). The monitor now shows ventricular fibrillation. The patient is pulseless and apneic. Your best course of action will be to:

   a. administer epinephrine, 1 mg (1:10,000) IV bolus

   b. administer a synchronized countershock with 100J

   c. begin CPR, intubate at once and establish IV access

   d. assure the synchronizer switch is off and immediately defibrillate with 200J

4. A 53 year old male is complaining of palpitations. He denies chest pain or difficulty breathing. His initial blood pressure is 128/64, his pulse 88 and regular. You have attached the monitor leads to the patient's chest and note a wide QRS-complex tachycardia. Recommended treatment guidelines for this patient include:

   a. O_2, IV, attempt vagal maneuvers and administer verapamil 2.5 mg IV bolus

   b. O_2, IV, administer sedation and deliver an unsynchronized countershock with 50J

   c. O_2, IV, administer an IV bolus of lidocaine, 1-1.5 mg/kg and reassess the patient

   d. O_2, IV, administer sedation and deliver a series of "stacked" synchronized countershocks with 100-200-300-360J

5. A 73 year old male is found pulseless and apneic. CPR is initiated. The cardiac monitor shows ventricular fibrillation. The proper energy levels for delivery of the initial "stacked" shocks to this patient would be:

   a. 50, 100, 200J
   b. 100, 200, 360J
   c. 100, 200, 300J
   d. 200, 200-300, 360J

6.

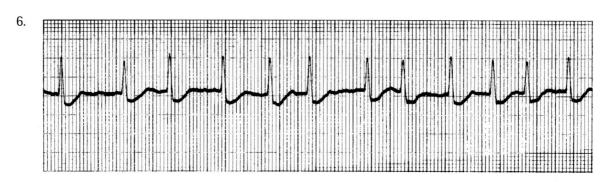

Figure 7-3

The rhythm shown above is:_____

7. When the adhesive pads of the automated external defibrillator (AED) have been attached:

   a. CPR should be continued while the analysis control button is pressed
   b. all contact with the patient must cease when the device is placed in analysis mode
   c. assessment of the rhythm takes approximately 60-90 seconds, depending on the brand of AED
   d. the device will announce that a shock is indicated if asystole is present by a written message, visual alarm or voice-synthesized statement

8. Synchronized countershock:

   a. is used only for atrial dysrhythmias
   b. delivers a shock between the peak and end of the T wave
   c. is used only for rhythms with a ventricular response of < 60/minute
   d. delivers a shock a few milliseconds after the highest part of the R wave

9. A 56 year old male has a permanent pacemaker in place. Should it be necessary to defibrillate this patient, conventional defibrillator paddles should be placed:

   a. directly over the pacemaker generator
   b. 5 inches from the pacemaker generator
   c. 6-12 inches from the pacemaker generator
   d. it makes no difference where the paddles are placed

10. Which of the following best describes an idioventricular (ventricular escape rhythm)?

   a. rapid, chaotic rhythm with no pattern or regularity
   b. gradual alteration in the amplitude and direction of the QRS; atrial rate indiscernible, ventricular rate 150-250 beats/minute
   c. essentially regular ventricular rhythm with QRS complexes measuring >.12; atrial rate not discernible; ventricular rate 20-40 beats/minute
   d. regular ventricular rhythm with QRS complexes measuring <.10; P waves may occur before, during or after the QRS; ventricular rate 40-60 beats/minute

11. Emergent transcutaneous pacing is indicated in all of the following situations EXCEPT:

   a. ventricular fibrillation
   b. complete heart block
   c. permanent pacemaker failure
   d. symptomatic second degree heart block

12. The precordial thump:

   1. is contraindicated in infants and children
   2. should never be allowed to delay defibrillation
   3. is a BLS technique that can and should be taught to lay rescuers
   4. should never initiated in a patient in VT with a pulse unless a defibrillator and pacemaker are immediately available

   a. 1, 2
   b. 2, 3
   c. 1, 2, 4
   d. 1, 3, 4

Questions 19-21 refer to the following scenario.

A pulseless and apneic 34 year old male is brought by ambulance to your busy Emergency Department. Basic EMTs report the patient was shot multiple times in the chest and abdomen with a large-caliber handgun. Chest compressions are being performed and the patient is being ventilated with a bag-valve device. An oropharyngeal airway is in place. The cardiac monitor displays the following rhythm:

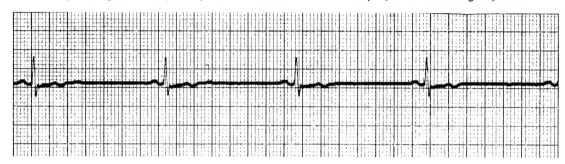

Figure 7-5

19. The rhythm displayed above is _____

20. The patient is unconscious, pulseless and apneic. This clinical situation is termed:

   a. asystole
   b. ventricular fibrillation
   c. idioventricular rhythm
   d. pulseless electrical activity.

21. List five (5) possible causes of the clinical situation presented above.

   1. _____

   2. _____

   3. _____

   4. _____

   5. _____

22. Medications that might be administered in this situation include:

   a. atropine and bretylium
   b. bretylium and lidocaine
   c. epinephrine and atropine
   d. lidocaine and epinephrine

23. Synchronized countershock may be used for all of the following EXCEPT:

    a. torsades de pointes, unstable patient, sustained rhythm
    b. ventricular tachycardia, unstable patient
    c. paroxysmal supraventricular tachycardia, unstable patient
    d. atrial fibrillation with a rapid ventricular response, unstable patient

24. The inherent rate of the ventricles is:

    a. 20-40 beats/minute
    b. 40-60 beats/minute
    c. 60-100 beats/minute
    d. 100-180 beats/minute

25. The difference between second degree type I and type II AV block is that with:

    a. type I the P waves occur irregularly
    b. type I the ventricular rhythm is regular
    c. type II the PR interval is always less than .12 seconds in duration
    d. type I the PR interval becomes progressively longer until a P wave appears without a QRS complex

26. The term used for three or more premature ventricular complexes (PVCs) occurring sequentially is:

    a. ventricular bigeminy
    b. ventricular fibrillation
    c. a run of ventricular tachycardia
    d. a run of ventricular escape beats

Questions 27 and 28 refer to the following scenario.

A 73 year old, 70 kg, female presents with a sudden onset of chest pain, dizziness and nausea. She has a long history of coronary artery disease and suffered an MI 8 months ago. Daily medications include Lanoxin and Furosemide. Her blood pressure is 54/32, respirations 12/minute. A weak pulse is present. The cardiac monitor reveals the following rhythm:

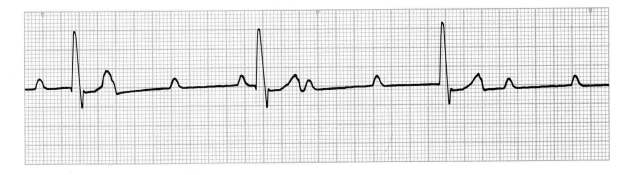

Figure 7-6   (Reproduced with permission from Huszar. RJ: *Basic dysrhythmias: interpretation and management,* 2/e, St. Louis, 1994, Mosby-Year Book, Inc.)

27. The rhythm shown is_____

28. Treatment for this patient should include:

    a. O_2, IV, lidocaine 1-1.5 mg/kg
    b. O_2, IV, epinephrine 1 mg IV bolus
    c. O_2, IV, morphine 1-3 mg, dopamine infusion at 5-20 µg/kg/min
    d. O_2, IV, transcutaneous pacing until a transvenous pacer can be placed

29. Select the correct statement(s) regarding defibrillation.

    1. Transthoracic resistance is significantly reduced when defibrillation is performed on a patient's bare skin.
    2. A patient should not be defibrillated more than four times in any one resuscitation effort.
    3. When delivering the three initial shocks for a patient in VF or pulseless VT, the paddles should be removed from the patient's chest and a pulse checked between each shock.
    4. The longer VF persists, the less likely electrical defibrillation will succeed.

    a. 4
    b. 1, 3
    c. 1, 2
    d. 2, 3, 4

30. Label the correct position for electrode placement for monitoring of Lead III.

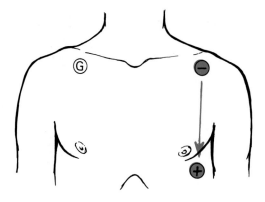

Figure 7-7

31. Defibrillation:
    a. "jump-starts" the heart
    b. increases coronary circulation and myocardial perfusion
    c. requires depressing the buttons on both defibrillator paddles in order to deliver a shock
    d. requires the presence of a clearly identifiable QRS before the machine will allow a discharge of energy

32.

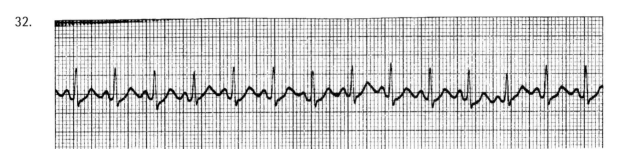

Figure 7-8

The rhythm shown above is_____

33.

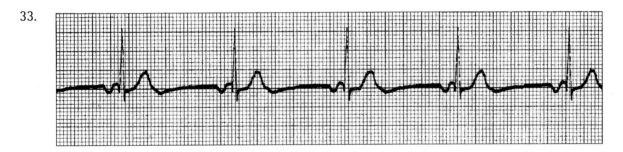

Figure 7-9

The rhythm shown above is_____

Questions 34–35 refer to the following scenario.

Your patient is a 38 year old female complaining of "fluttering" in her chest. Although she denies chest pain, she appears quite apprehensive. Her skin is pale, cool and dry. Breath sounds are clear bilaterally. BP 114/64, R 24 and nonlabored. The ECG is as follows:

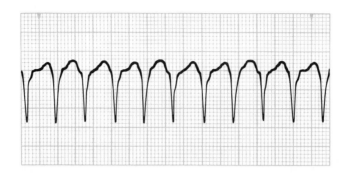

Figure 7-10   (Reproduced with permission from Huszar. RJ: *Basic dysrhythmias: interpretation and management,* 2/e, St. Louis, 1994, Mosby-Year Book, Inc.)

34. The rhythm shown above is_____

35. Recommended treatment guidelines for this patient would include:

   a. O$_2$, IV, prophylactic lidocaine 1 mg/kg IV bolus
   b. O$_2$, IV, vagal maneuvers, adenosine 6 mg rapid IV bolus
   c. O$_2$, IV, vagal maneuvers, verapamil 2.5 mg slow IV bolus
   d. O$_2$, IV, administer sedation and perform synchronized countershock with 50J

36.

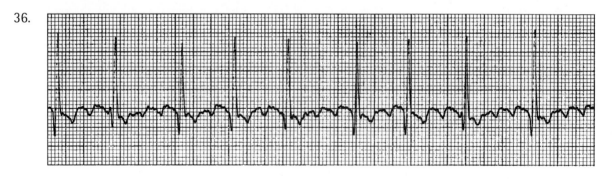

Figure 7-11

   The rhythm shown above is_____

37. Select the INCORRECTLY matched patient situation and rhythm with the recommended energy settings.

    a. polymorphic VT, sustained rhythm, unstable patient: unsynchronized countershock with 200, 200-300, 360J

    b. ventricular fibrillation: unsynchronized countershock with 200, 200-300, 360J

    c. atrial fibrillation with a rapid ventricular response, unstable patient: synchronized countershock with 100-200-300-360J

    d. atrial flutter with a rapid ventricular response, unstable patient: unsynchronized countershock with 100-200-300-360J

38.

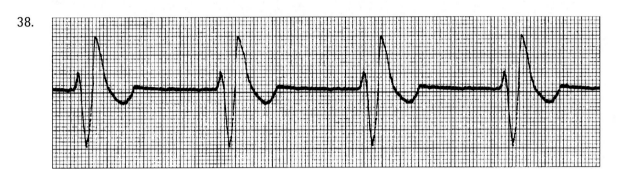

Figure 7-12

The rhythm shown above is_____

39. The period of time in which no amount of stimulus can produce early depolarization is referred to as the:

    a. resting state
    b. early recovery period
    c. absolute refractory period
    d. relative refractory period

Questions 40-41 refer to the following scenario.

A 54 year old male is complaining of severe midsternal chest pain radiating to his jaw and "skipped beats". He states the pain has been present for approximately 1 hour and has not been relieved with rest. He has no significant past medical history. BP 136/84, R 12/minute. Your monitor displays the following rhythm:

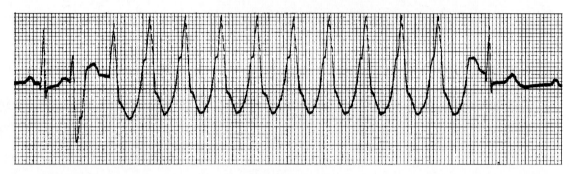

Figure 7-13

40.   The rhythm shown above is _____

41.   Interventions which should be considered in the management of this patient include:

    a. O$_2$, IV, lidocaine 1.5 mg/kg

    b. O$_2$, IV, atropine 0.5 mg every 3-5 minutes to a maximum of 0.03 mg/kg

    c. O$_2$, IV, nitroglycerin, morphine 1-3 mg titrated to pain relief, lidocaine bolus and maintenance infusion, aspirin and thrombolytic therapy

    d. O$_2$, IV, administer sedation and perform synchronized countershock with 50J

42.   A condition in which progression of an electrical impulse is delayed, blocked (or both) in one or more portions of the electrical conduction system while the electrical impulse is conducted normally through the rest of the conduction system best describes:

    a. reentry

    b. automaticity

    c. the vulnerable period

    d. the absolute refractory period

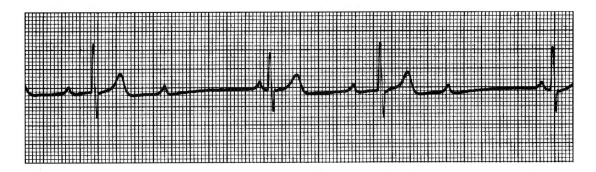

Figure 7-14

43. The rhythm shown above is: _____

44. Depolarization is the same as contraction.

    a. true

    b. false

45. Label the absolute and relative refractory periods on the figure below.

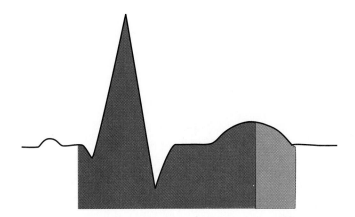

Figure 7-15

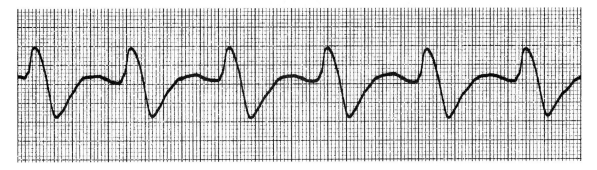

Figure 7-16

46. The rhythm shown above is: _____

47. Select the INCORRECT statement regarding a complete (third-degree) AV block.

    a. in complete AV block, the atrial rate is greater than the ventricular rate
    b. in complete AV block, the atria and ventricles beat independently of each other
    c. in complete AV block, the ventricular rhythm is essentially regular although the P waves occur irregularly
    d. in complete AV block, the QRS may be either wide or narrow, depending on the origin of the escape pacemaker

48. The rhythm shown below is: _____

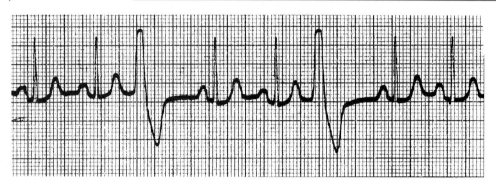

Figure 7-17

49. The rhythm shown below is: _____

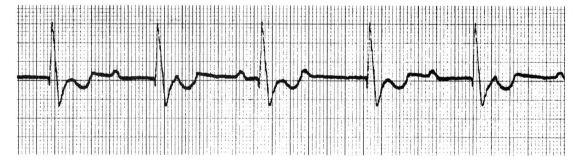

Figure 7-18

50. The rhythm shown below is: _____

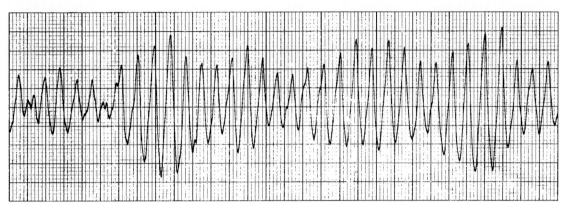

Figure 7-19

MONITORING AND DYSRHYTHMIA RECOGNITION/ ELECTRICAL THERAPY QUIZ ANSWERS

QUESTION	ANSWER	RATIONALE	JAMA PAGE REFERENCE
1	D	The AED delivers a shock by means of two adhesive pads applied to the patient: upper-right sternal border, lower-left ribs over the cardiac apex.	N/A
2	B	Sinus arrhythmia is a normal rhythm seen in children and physically fit adults. The rhythm is phasic with respiration: Inspiration → increased rate, expiration → decreased rate.	N/A
3	D	Assure the synchronizer switch is off and immediately defibrillate with 200J.	2212
4	C	This patient is clinically stable. Administer oxygen, establish an IV, and administer an IV bolus of lidocaine 1-1.5 mg/kg.	2223
5	D	The initial energy levels for the three stacked shocks in pulseless VT/VF are 200J, 200-300J and 360J.	2216
6		The rhythm shown is atrial fibrillation with an irregular ventricular response.	N/A
7	B	When the AED is placed in analysis mode, all contact with the patient must cease.	N/A
8	D	Synchronized countershock delivers a shock a few milliseconds after the highest part of the R wave.	2226
9	B	Defibrillator paddles should be placed 5 inches from the pacemaker generator.	N/A
10	C	"A" describes ventricular fibrillation. "B" describes torsade and "D" describes a junctional rhythm. An idioventricular (ventricular escape) rhythm is characterized by wide QRS complexes occurring at an essentially regular rate of 20-40 beats per minute.	N/A

11	A	Transcutaneous pacing is not indicated in ventricular fibrillation - defibrillation is the treatment of choice for VF.	2214
12	C	The precordial thump is an ACLS technique and should NOT be taught to lay rescuers.	2213
13	B	The AICD generator unit is found in the left upper quadrant of the patient's abdomen and takes approximately 10-35 seconds to sense VT or VF, charge its capacitors and deliver a shock. These devices are indicated for treatment of patient suffering from, or at risk for, sudden cardiac arrest. "D" refers to operation of a semi-automated *external* defibrillator.	N/A
14	A	The relative refractory period is also known as the vulnerable period.	N/A
15	B	Defibrillation is not indicated in pulseless electrical activity or asystole. Since electric shocks produce parasympathetic discharge, defibrillation may eliminate any possibility for return of spontaneous cardiac activity. Defibrillation is indicated in VF, the unstable patient with polymorphic VT, whenever there is a delay in synchronization of a rhythm or the patient's clinical condition is critical.	2220, 2224
16	D	Second-degree AV block, Type II is often associated with anteroseptal MI and may progress rapidly to a third degree (complete) AV block.	2222
17		The rhythm displayed is asystole. Continue CPR. Intubate at once (confirm tube placement), establish an IV of normal saline or lactated Ringer's solution, and confirm the rhythm in another lead. Consider possible causes of the arrest (hypoxia, hyperkalemia, hypokalemia, hypothermia, acidosis, drug overdose) and treat accordingly. Consider immediate transcutaneous pacing. Administer epinephrine 1 mg IV push (or 2-2$\frac{1}{2}$ mg via the endotracheal tube). Administer atropine 1 mg IV push (or 2-2$\frac{1}{2}$ mg via the endotracheal tube). Consider termination of efforts if no response.	2220

18	A	The dominant pacemaker of the heart is normally the sino-atrial (SA) node.	N/A
19		The rhythm displayed is a sinus bradycardia.	N/A
20	D	Despite the presence of the rhythm on the monitor, the patient is pulseless. This situation is termed pulseless electrical activity.	2219
21		Possible causes of pulseless electrical activity include (MATCHx4ED): • Myocardial infarction (massive acute) • Acidosis • Tension pneumothorax • Cardiac tamponade • Hypovolemia, Hypoxemia, • Hyperkalemia, Hypothermia • Embolism (massive pulmonary) • Drug overdose Of those listed, specific causes that should be immediately evaluated in this patient include acidosis, the presence of a tension pneumothorax and/or pericardial tamponade, hypovolemia and hypoxemia.	2219
22	C	Epinephrine and atropine may be administered in cases of pulseless electrical activity. Additional medications may also be administered based on the cause of PEA.	2219
23	A	Unsynchronized countershock (defibrillation) is indicated in the unstable patient in sustained torsade.	2220
24	A	The inherent rate of the ventricles is 20-40 beats/minute.	N/A
25	D	With second degree AV block, type I, the PR interval becomes progressively longer until a P wave is no longer conducted. The PR intervals in second degree AV block type II remain constant for each conducted QRS.	N/A
26	C	Three or more PVCs occurring sequentially are referred to as a salvo, burst or run of ventricular tachycardia.	N/A

27	B	The rhythm displayed has a regular ventricular rhythm and more P waves than QRS complexes. The P waves occur regularly. There is no association of the P waves to the QRS complexes, thus this rhythm is a complete (third-degree) AV block.	N/A
28	D	This complete block has a wide-QRS complex indicating a ventricular escape pacemaker. Administer oxygen, initiate an IV and initiate transcutaneous pacing while awaiting transvenous pacemaker placement. Epinephrine boluses are not administered to patients with a pulse. Lidocaine is not indicated and morphine should not be administered due to the patient's hypotension.	2221-2222
29	A	The longer VF persists, the less likely electrical defibrillation will succeed. It is necessary to apply defib pads to the patient's chest or gel to defibrillator paddles to reduce the resistance of the chest wall to current. There are no specific limitations as to the number of times a patient may be defibrillated during a resuscitation effort. Current AHA guidelines advocate leaving conventional defibrillator paddles on the chest when delivering the initial "stacked" shock sequence and not stopping to check pulses during the shock sequence unless a rhythm other than VF/VT appears on the screen.	2215-2217
30	Figure 7-20 Lead III.		N/A
31	C	Defibrillation requires depressing the buttons on both conventional defibrillator paddles in order to deliver a shock.	N/A

32		The rhythm shown is a sinus tachycardia with a ventricular response of approximately 150 beats/minute.	N/A
33		The dysrhythmia shown is a junctional rhythm. No P waves are seen; there is a narrow, regular QRS complex occurring at a regular rate of approximately 50 beats/minute.	N/A
34		The QRS measures less than 0.12 sec and occurs regularly. There are no P waves seen. The ventricular response is > 150/minute. This rhythm is a supraventricular tachycardia.	N/A
35	B	This patient is stable. Administer oxygen, initiate an IV, attempt vagal maneuvers, and administer adenosine 6 mg, rapid IV bolus.	2223
36		The rhythm displayed is atrial flutter.	
37	D	Atrial flutter with a rapid ventricular response, unstable patient should received synchronized countershock starting with 50 joules and increasing to 100-200-300 and 360J.	2224
38		The rhythm shown is an idioventricular (ventricular escape) rhythm. Wide QRS complexes are present occurring at a regular rate of 38 beats/minute.	N/A
39	C	The absolute refractory period corresponds with the onset of the QRS to the peak of the T wave. During this period, the myocardial working cells cannot contract and the cells of the electrical conduction system cannot conduct an electrical impulse - no matter how strong.	N/A
40		The rhythm shown is a sinus rhythm with a run of VT (three or more PVCs occurring sequentially are referred to as run of VT).	N/A

41	C	This patient is displaying signs and symptoms consistent with an acute MI. Administer O_2, initiate an IV, administer nitroglycerin. If no relief, or pain is severe, administer morphine 1-3 mg titrated to pain relief. Due to the presence of ventricular ectopy in the setting of an acute MI, administer a lidocaine bolus and initiate a maintenance infusion, administer aspirin and consider thrombolytic therapy.	2231
42	A	Reentry is a condition in which progression of an electrical impulse is delayed, blocked (or both) in one or more portions of the electrical conduction system while the electrical impulse is conducted normally through the rest of the conduction system.	N/A
43		The rhythm shown is a second degree AV block type I. The P waves occur regularly and the PR intervals lengthen until a P wave appears without a QRS.	N/A
44	B	Depolarization is **NOT** the same as contraction. Although depolarization is expected to result in contraction, this is not always the case - as in pulseless electrical activity.	2219
45	**Figure 7-21** Absolute and relative refractory periods		N/A
46		The rhythm shown is an accelerated idioventricular rhythm.	N/A

47	C	In complete AV block, the ventricular rhythm is essentially regular. There are more P waves than QRS complexes and the P wave occur regularly. The QRS may be wide or narrow depending on the origin of the escape pacemaker. The PR intervals are completely variable as the atria and ventricles beat independently of each other.	N/A
48		The rhythm shown is sinus tachycardia with ventricular trigeminy.	N/A
49		The rhythm shown is complete (third-degree) AV block. There are more P waves than QRS complexes, the P waves occur regularly, the ventricular rhythm is regular, and the PR intervals are completely variable.	N/A
50	D	The rhythm shown is Torsades de Pointes.	N/A

Cardiovascular Pharmacology

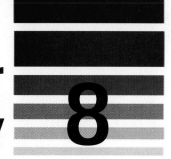

8

Objectives

Upon completion of this chapter, you will be able to:

1. Describe the location and effects of stimulation of α, β and dopaminergic receptors.

2. Define the following terms:
   - Afterload
   - Agonist
   - Antagonist
   - Chronotrope
   - Dromotrope
   - Inotrope
   - Parasympatholytic
   - Preload
   - Sympathomimetic

3. Identify the primary neurotransmitter for the sympathetic and parasympathetic divisions of the autonomic nervous system.

4. Identify the mechanism of action, indications, dosage and precautions for each of the following medications:
   - Oxygen
   - Nitroglycerin
   - Morphine sulfate
   - Lidocaine
   - Procainamide
   - Bretylium
   - β-blockers
   - Calcium channel blockers
   - Atropine
   - Isoproterenol
   - Verapamil
   - Adenosine
   - Magnesium sulfate
   - Calcium chloride
   - Epinephrine
   - Norepinephrine
   - Dopamine
   - Dobutamine
   - Amrinone
   - Sodium nitroprusside
   - Sodium bicarbonate
   - Furosemide
   - Thrombolytic agents

TABLE 8-1.   REVIEW OF THE AUTONOMIC NERVOUS SYSTEM.

	SYMPATHETIC DIVISION	PARASYMPATHETIC DIVISION
	"Fight or Flight" response • Mobilizes the body • Allows the body to function under stress	"Feed and Breed" response • Conservation of body resources • Restoration of body resources
Receptors	**Alpha (α)-1** _peripheral arterioles_ • Located in vascular smooth muscle • Stimulation results in vasoconstriction **Alpha (α)-2** • Located in skeletal blood vessels • Inhibits the release of norepinephrine **Beta (β)-1 (one heart)** _Myocardium_ • Located in the heart _SA node AV node_ • Stimulation results in heart rate, ↑ conduction, ↑ contractility **Beta (β)-2 (two lungs)** • Located in the smooth muscle of the bronchi and the skeletal blood vessels _arterioles; Lungs_ • Stimulation results in relaxation of the bronchi and vasodilation **Dopaminergic** • Located in the coronary arteries, renal, mesenteric and visceral blood vessels • Stimulation results in dilation _↑ renal + mesenteric blood flow_	**Nicotinic** receptors located in skeletal muscle. **Muscarinic** receptors located in smooth muscle. Organs and the effects of parasympathetic stimulation: Bronchi • Stimulation results in constriction, ↑ secretion Eye • Pupillary constriction Salivary glands • ↑ salivation Heart • ↓ heart rate GI tract • ↑ secretions, ↑ peristalsis
Neurotransmitter	Epinephrine, norepinephrine	Acetylcholine
Synonymous terms	Adrenergic, sympathomimetic, catecholamine, anticholinergic, parasympatholytic, cholinergic blocker	Cholinergic, parasympathomimetic, sympathetic blocker, cholinomimetic, sympatholytic, adrenergic blocker
Opposite terms	Sympatholytic, antiadrenergic, sympathetic blocker, adrenergic blocker	Parasympatholytic, anticholinergic, cholinergic blocker, vagolytic

TERMS TO REMEMBER	
Inotrope	A substance which affects myocardial contractility • Positive inotrope = ↑ force of contraction • Negative inotrope = ↓ force of contraction
Chronotrope	A substance which affects the heart rate • Positive chronotrope = ↑ heart rate • Negative chronotrope = ↓ heart rate
Dromotrope	A substance which affects AV conduction velocity • Positive dromotrope = ↑ AV conduction velocity • Negative dromotrope = ↓ AV conduction velocity
Preload	The pressure/volume in the left ventricle at the end of diastole
Afterload	The pressure or resistance against which the heart must pump
Agonist	A drug or substance that produces a predictable response (stimulates action)
Antagonist	An agent that exerts an opposite action to another (blocks action)

DRUGS USED FOR MYOCARDIAL ISCHEMIA/PAIN

DRUG	MECHANISM OF ACTION/EFFECTS	INDICATIONS	DOSAGE	PRECAUTIONS
Oxygen	• $\uparrow$ O_2 tension • $\uparrow$ hemoglobin saturation if ventilation is supported • Improves tissue oxygenation when circulation is maintained	Highest possible O_2 concentration (preferably 100%) should be administered as soon as possible to all patients with: • ischemic chest pain • cardiac or pulmonary arrest • suspected hypoxemia of any cause	In the spontaneously breathing patient: • Nasal cannula (1-6 liters/min) • Simple mask (6-10 liters/min) In cardiac arrest: positive pressure ventilation with 100% oxygen	Toxicity with prolonged administration of high flow oxygen - rarely a concern in the emergent situation Obstructive lung disease • Do not withhold oxygen if signs of hypoxia present • Be prepared to intubate and assist ventilation as necessary
Nitroglycerin **Class:** Organic nitrate, Vasodilator, Antianginal **Trade Name(s):** Nitrostat, Nitrobid (SL forms) Tridil (IV)	• Smooth muscle relaxant $\rightarrow$ $\downarrow$ venous return (preload) $\rightarrow$ $\downarrow$ ventricular volume $\rightarrow$ $\downarrow$ ventricular work $\rightarrow$ $\uparrow$ perfusion • Peripheral vasodilation $\rightarrow$ $\downarrow$ afterload $\rightarrow$ $\downarrow$ ventricular work • Coronary artery vasodilation • Heart rate may $\uparrow$ as a result of $\downarrow$ blood pressure	**Sublingual:** • Ischemic chest pain • Cardiogenic pulmonary edema **IV:** • Unstable angina • CHF associated with MI	**Sublingual:** 0.3 or 0.4 mg repeated at 5 minute intervals to maximum of 3 doses **IV infusion:** Mix 50 mg in 250 ml (200 μg/ml) Continuous infusion starting at 10-20 μg/min and $\uparrow$ by 5-10 μg/min every 5-10 min until the desired hemodynamic or clinical response occurs	Primary side effect is hypotension • Monitor blood pressure closely before, during and after administration • Hypotension may exacerbate myocardial ischemia • Responds readily to fluid replacement therapy Other side effects include: • Tachycardia (thought to be due to $\downarrow$ blood pressure) • Paradoxical bradycardia • Headache • Reperfusion dysrhythmias • Palpitations
Morphine Sulfate **Class:** Narcotic Analgesic	• $\uparrow$ venous capacitance (pools blood in the periphery) • $\downarrow$ venous return (preload) • $\downarrow$ systemic vascular resistance (afterload) • $\downarrow$ myocardial oxygen demand • $\uparrow$ pain threshold	Ischemic chest pain (Pain $\uparrow$ sympathetic response$\rightarrow$$\uparrow$heart rate, $\uparrow$ systemic vascular resistance,$\uparrow$ blood pressure $\rightarrow$$\uparrow$ myocardial O_2 consumption = pain relief is a **priority** in the management of these patients) Acute pulmonary edema	1-3 mg slowly IV bolus every 5 minutes titrated to desired analgesic or hemodynamic effect Onset: IV = immediate Peak: IV = 20 minutes	Watch closely for: Respiratory depression, bradycardia, CNS depression, nausea/ vomiting, systemic hypotension - especially in patients with volume depletion Reversible with naloxone (Narcan)

DRUGS USED FOR HEART RHYTHM AND RATE

DRUG	MECHANISM OF ACTION/EFFECTS	INDICATIONS	DOSAGE	PRECAUTIONS
Lidocaine Hydrochloride **Trade Name:** Xylocaine **Class:** Ventricular antidysrhythmic	• Suppresses ventricular ectopy • ↑ VF threshold • Does not significantly affect myocardial contractility in therapeutic doses	• Significant ventricular ectopy (runs of VT, "R on T" PVCs) seen in the setting of acute MI/ischemia • VT/VF that persist after defibrillation and administration of epinephrine • VT with a pulse • Wide-complex tachycardia of uncertain origin **Routine prophylactic use in uncomplicated MI or ischemia without PVCs is no longer recommended**	**VF/Pulseless VT:** 1-1.5 mg/kg repeated in 5-10 min to maximum dose of 3 mg/kg **VT with pulse/Wide-complex tachycardia of uncertain origin, significant ventricular ectopy (PVCs):** 1-1.5 mg/kg repeated every 5-10 min as needed with 0.5-0.75 mg/kg to total dose of 3 mg/kg **Only bolus therapy used in cardiac arrest** After return of pulse, continuous infusion (IV drip): after 1 mg/kg → drip 2 mg/min after $1^1/_2$-2 mg/kg → drip 3 mg/min after $2^1/_2$-3 mg/kg → drip 4 mg/min **To mix drip:** 1 gram in 250 ml or 2 grams in 500 ml. Using a microdrip (60 gtts/ml) administration set: 1 mg/min = 15 gtts/min 2 mg/min = 30 gtts/min 3 mg/min = 45 gtts/min 4 mg/min = 60 gtts/min Endotracheal dose 2 - $2^1/_2$ times IV dose diluted in 10 ml normal saline or distilled water	Indications of toxicity are usually CNS related: • muscle twitching • seizures • slurred speech • altered LOC Because lidocaine is metabolized in the liver, reduce dose in: • decreased cardiac output (acute MI, CHF, shock) • elderly patients (>70 years) • hepatic dysfunction In these patients, the normal bolus dose should be administered first, followed by $^1/_2$ the normal maintenance infusion Do not treat ventricular ectopy first if the heart rate is < 60 beats/minute - treat the bradycardia **Lidocaine may be lethal in a bradycardia with a ventricular escape rhythm (second degree AV block, type II, third-degree (complete) AV block with a wide-QRS**[1]

DRUG	MECHANISM OF ACTION/EFFECTS	INDICATIONS	DOSAGE	PRECAUTIONS
Procainamide **Trade Name:** Pronestyl **Class:** Antidysrhythmic	• Suppresses ventric-ular ectopy • ↑ VF threshold • Shortens effective refractory period of the AV node • Prolongs effective refractory period and duration of the action potential in the His-Purkinje system	Recommended when lidocaine is con-traindicated or has failed to suppress ventricular ectopy • Wide-complex tachycardias that cannot be distin-guished from VT (not a first-line drug) • Atrial fibrillation with a rapid ven-tricular response (not a first-line drug) • Suppression of recurrent VT that cannot be con-trolled with lido-caine • Refractory pulseless VT/VF	IV infusion of 100 mg over 5 minutes (20 mg/min) until one of the following occurs: • **dysrhythmia is suppressed** • **QRS widens by 50% of its original width** • **hypotension devel-ops** • **total of 17 mg/kg has been adminis-tered (1.2 gm for a 70 kg patient)** Note: up to 30 mg/min may be administered in urgent situations To prepare infusion: Mix 1 gram/250 ml or 2 grams/500 ml (4 mg/ml) Maintenance infusion is 1-4 mg/min	• ↓ maintenance infusion in renal failure, CHF or liver dysfunction • Hypotension may occur if injected too rapidly - use cau-tiously in patients with acute MI • Avoid in patients with pre-existing QT prolongation and torsades de pointes • Observe ECG for ↑ PR and QT intervals, widening QRS and heart block

DRUG	MECHANISM OF ACTION/EFFECTS	INDICATIONS	DOSAGE	PRECAUTIONS
Bretylium Tosylate **Trade Name:** Bretylol **Class:** Ventricular anti-dysrhythmic, Adrenergic blocker	Initial sympath-omimetic effects due to release of norepi-nephrine: • ↑ heart rate • ↑ peripheral vaso-constriction • ↑ blood pressure • ↑ cardiac output Subsequent sympa-tholytic response after 15-20 minutes (adrenergic block): • ↓ blood pressure • Suppresses ventric-ular ectopy • ↑ VF threshold	Not a first-line anti-dysrhythmic • After defibrillation, epinephrine and lidocaine have failed to convert VF • VF has recurred despite epinephrine and lidocaine • Lidocaine and pro-cainamide have failed to control VT associated with a pulse • Lidocaine and adenosine have failed to control wide-complex tachycardias	**Refractory VF/pulse-less VT:** 5 mg/kg rapid IV **bolus** followed by defibrillation If VF persists, ↑ dose to 10 mg/kg and repeat every 5 min to maximum dose 30-35 mg/kg If conversion occurs to a perfusing rhythm after bolus therapy, initiate a continuous infusion at 1-2 mg/min To mix drip: 1 gram in 250 ml or 2 grams in 500 ml. Using a microdrip (60 gtts/ml) administration set: 1 mg/min = 15 gtts/min 2 mg/min = 30 gtts/min **Persistently recurring VT (with a pulse):** **(IV infusion)** 5-10 mg/kg diluted in 50 ml and infused over 8-10 min to avoid nausea/vomiting. Repeat dose 5-10 mg/kg in 1-2 hours.	Postural hypotension Nausea/vomiting with rapid IV administra-tion Contraindicated in digitalis toxicity Additive effects with sympathomimetics

DRUG	MECHANISM OF ACTION/EFFECTS	INDICATIONS	DOSAGE	PRECAUTIONS
β-Adrenergic Blockers Atenolol (Tenormin) Esmolol (Brevibloc) Metoprolol (Lopressor) Propranolol (Inderal)	β-adrenergic receptor blockade Competitive with adrenergic stimulants Action depends on level of adrenergic influence Antidysrhythmic (quinidine) effect	↓ incidence of VF in post-MI patients who did not receive thrombolytic agents When used within 4 hours after administration of thrombolytic therapy, may ↓ rate of nonfatal reinfarction and recurrent ischemia In thrombolytic treated patients, may ↓ mortality and recurrent MI if administered within 2 hours of symptom onset	Atenolol: 5-10 mg IV over 5 min Esmolol: 500 μg/kg over 1 minute (loading dose) followed by a maintenance infusion at 50 μg/kg/min over 4 minutes Metoprolol: 5-10 mg slow IV push at 5 min intervals to total of 15 mg Propranolol: Total dose of 0.1 mg/kg slow IV push divided into 3 equal doses at 2-3 in intervals	Should be avoided in: • bradycardia • second or third-degree AV block • hypotension • overt CHF • lung disease associated with bronchospasm
Atropine Sulfate Class: Anticholinergic (Parasympathetic blocker) Antidysrhythmic	Parasympathetic blocking (vagolytic) action: • ↑ heart rate (↑ sinus node discharge) • Improves AV conduction • May restore cardiac rhythm in asystole (if asystole due to ↑ parasympathetic tone, atropine may reverse effects → restore rhythm)	Symptomatic: • Sinus bradycardia • Junctional escape rhythm • Second-degree AV block, type I • Third-degree AV block with narrow QRS (junctional escape pacer) Class IIB (possibly helpful) in AV block at the His-Purkinje level (type II AV block and third-degree AV block with new wide-QRS complexes)[2] • Asystole • Bradycardiac pulseless electrical activity	Asystole/Pulseless Electrical Activity: 1.0 mg IV every 3-5 min to maximum dose of 3 mg Symptomatic Bradycardia: 0.5-1.0 mg repeated every 3-5 min to max dose 2-3 mg Endotracheal dose 2-2$^1/_2$ times IV dose diluted in 10 ml normal saline or distilled water	• Administer oxygen prior to administration of atropine • Should not be pushed slowly or in doses of < 0.5 mg as a paradoxical bradycardia may occur • Use with caution in the setting of acute MI. As atropine ↑ heart rate → ↑ myocardial O_2 demand → worsened ischemia → may ↑ zone of infarction • 3 mg considered the vagolytic dose (total vagal nerve inhibition) in most patients

DRUG	MECHANISM OF ACTION/EFFECTS	INDICATIONS	DOSAGE	PRECAUTIONS
Isoproterenol **Trade Name:** Isuprel **Class:** Sympathomimetic, Beta-Agonist, Synthetic Catecholamine	Pure β-adrenergic stimulator (β-1 and β-2) • Potent chronotropic effect (heart rate) (**primary** effect) • Inotropic effect ($\uparrow$ force of contraction) • $\uparrow$ cardiac output • myocardial O_2 consumption $\rightarrow \uparrow$ myocardial ischemia • Vasodilation	Class IIa (probably helpful) Refractory torsades de pointes (shortens the QT interval and prevents bradycardia which may precipitate torsade) Class IIb (possibly helpful) in low doses for symptomatic bradycardia (after atropine, pacing, dopamine and epinephrine) Class III (may be harmful) in higher doses for symptomatic bradycardia	2-10 μg/min titrated to desired response (for bradycardia, usually titrated to a heart rate of 60 beats/minute) To mix drip: 1 mg in 250 ml (4 μg/ml)	• If used for symptomatic bradycardia, should be used with extreme caution • Not indicated in patients with cardiac arrest or hypotension • Excessive tachycardia • Dysrhythmias • $\uparrow$ myocardial O_2 consumption
Verapamil **Trade Name(s):** Isoptin, Calan **Class:** Calcium channel blocker	• Slows conduction and $\uparrow$ refractoriness in the AV node • May terminate reentrant dysrhythmias that require AV nodal conduction for their continuation • May control ventricular response in patients with atrial fibrillation, atrial flutter or multifocal atrial tachycardia • May $\downarrow$ myocardial contractility • May exacerbate CHF in patients with severe left ventricular dysfunction	Narrow-complex PSVT (adenosine drug of choice) Atrial fibrillation or atrial flutter with a rapid ventricular response Wide-complex tachycardia known with certainty to be supraventricular in origin	2.5-5.0 mg slow IV bolus over 2 minutes. If no response, may repeat with 5-10 mg every 15-30 minutes to a maximum of 20 mg (if blood pressure normal or elevated).	• Avoid or use with caution in left ventricular dysfunction • Observe for hypotension • Avoid in patients with AV block, sinus node dysfunction or severe cardiac failure • Do not use in WPW with atrial fibrillation/flutter

DRUG	MECHANISM OF ACTION/EFFECTS	INDICATIONS	DOSAGE	PRECAUTIONS
Diltiazem **Trade Name:** Cardizem **Class:** Calcium channel blocker	• Slows conduction and increases refractoriness in the AV node • May terminate reentrant dysrhythmias that require AV nodal conduction for their continuation • May control ventricular response in patients with atrial fibrillation, atrial flutter or multifocal atrial tachycardia • May decrease myocardial contractility • May exacerbate CHF in patients with severe left ventricular dysfunction	Multifocal atrial tachycardia, atrial fibrillation or atrial flutter with a rapid ventricular response	0.25 mg/kg (20 mg) IV over 2 min followed 15 minutes later by 0.35 mg/kg (25 mg) IV over 2 minutes In atrial fibrillation with a rapid ventricular response, diltiazem may be used as a maintenance infusion of 5-15 mg/hour	• Produces less myocardial depression than verapamil • Avoid or use with caution in left ventricular dysfunction • Common side effects include hypotension and flushing • Avoid in patients with AV block, sinus node dysfunction or severe cardiac failure • Do not administer to patients with WPW - may worsen dysrhythmia • Not effective in VT
Adenosine **Trade Name:** Adenocard **Class:** Endogenous chemical, Antidysrhythmic	• ↓ sinus rate • ↓ conduction through AV node • Can interrupt reentrant pathways through the AV node • Has a direct effect on supraventricular tissue • Half-life is less than 5 seconds	• Conversion of supraventricular tachycardia to a regular sinus rhythm, including PSVT associated with accessory bypass tracts that involve the AV node (as seen in WPW) that is refractory to vagal maneuvers • Wide-complex tachycardia of uncertain type **after** lidocaine administration If the dysrhythmia is not due to reentry involving the AV node or sinus node (atrial fibrillation, atrial flutter, atrial or ventricular tachycardias), adenosine will not terminate the dysrhythmia but may produce transient AV block that may clarify the diagnosis	Initial bolus = 6 mg rapid IV bolus over 1-3 seconds followed by a 20 ml saline flush. Wait 1-2 minutes. If no response observed, administer 12 mg (may repeat the 12 mg dose once in 1-2 minutes) Due to extremely short half-life, start IV line as proximal to the heart as possible, such as the antecubital fossa. Onset: Seconds Peak: Seconds Duration: 10-12 seconds	Side effects common but transient and usually resolve spontaneously within 1-2 minutes - flushing, dyspnea, chest pain. Consider ↑ dose in patients on theophylline since methylxanthines prevent binding of adenosine at receptor sites Consider ↓ dose in patients on dipyridamole (Persantine) because adenosine potentiates its effects. Relatively high incidence of recurrence of the tachycardia after 6 mg dose; 92% conversion to a sinus rhythm after 12 mg bolus.

DRUG	MECHANISM OF ACTION/EFFECTS	INDICATIONS	DOSAGE	PRECAUTIONS
Magnesium Sulfate	May ↓ early MI mortality May ↓ incidence of dysrhythmias that often occur in survivors of MI Mechanism of action not completely understood. May ↓ mortality due to:[3] • systemic vasodilation → ↓ myocardial oxygen demand • ↓ platelet aggregation • coronary vasodilation • improved myocardial metabolism • ↓ myocardial infarct size • protection against catecholamine induced myocardial necrosis	Torsades de Pointes Pulseless VT/VF Acute MI Hypomagnesemia	**Pulseless VT/VF:** 1-2 grams IV (2-4 ml of 50% solution) diluted in 10 ml and administered over 1-2 minutes **Acute MI, Hypomagnesemia** Loading dose of 1-2 grams mixed in 50-100 ml and administered over 5-60 minutes **Torsades de Pointes** 1-2 grams IV (2-4 ml of 50% solution) diluted in 10 ml administered over 1-2 minutes followed by the same amount (mixed in 50-100 ml) infused over 1 hour	• Magnesium deficiency is associated with cardiac dysrhythmias, symptoms of cardiac insufficiency and sudden cardiac death • Signs/symptoms of magnesium overdose include ↓ respiratory rate, hypotension, hyporeflexia • Calcium chloride should be on hand for IV administration if signs of magnesium overdose develop

DRUGS USED TO IMPROVE CARDIAC OUTPUT AND BLOOD PRESSURE

DRUG	MECHANISM OF ACTION/EFFECTS	INDICATIONS	DOSAGE	PRECAUTIONS
Epinephrine **Trade Name:** Adrenalin **Class:** Sympathomimetic, Natural Catecholamine	Produces beneficial effects in patients during cardiac arrest primarily because of its α-**adrenergic** stimulating properties α-**adrenergic effects:** ↑ systemic vascular resistance (vasoconstriction) → ↑ diastolic pressure → ↑ myocardial and cerebral blood flow during CPR β-**adrenergic effects:** ↑ heart rate (+ chronotropy) ↑ myocardial contractility (+ inotropy) Results in ↑ myocardial oxygen demand	First agent in cardiac arrest: **IV BOLUS** • VF • Pulseless VT • Pulseless electrical activity • Asystole **INFUSION** • VF • Pulseless VT • Vasopressor agent for patients with symptomatic bradycardia (not a first-line agent)	1 mg of 1:10,000 solution IV bolus every 3-5 min **Intermediate dose:** 2-5 mg IV bolus every 3-5 min **Escalating dose:** 1 mg, 3 mg, 5 mg IV bolus (3 min apart) **High dose:** 0.1 mg/kg IV bolus every 3-5 min Epinephrine **infusion:** start at 1 μg/min and titrate to desired response (2-10 μg/min) To prepare infusion: mix 1 mg in 250 ml (4 μg/ml) Endotracheal dose 2-2$^1/_2$ times IV dose (prepare 2-2$^1/_2$ mg of epinephrine 1:1000 solution, add normal saline for total volume of 10 ml and administer)	• Continuous IV infusions of epinephrine should be administered via a central vein to the ↓ risk of extravasation • Should not be administered in the same IV line as alkaline solutions - inactivates epinephrine • Epinephrine infusion should be administered via an infusion pump
Norepinephrine **Trade Name:** Levophed **Class:** Sympathomimetic, Natural catecholamine	Naturally occurring potent vasoconstrictor (α-receptor stimulating agent) and inotropic (β-1 receptor stimulator) agent 90% α, 10% β· α activity usually dominant Usually causes renal and mesenteric vasoconstriction	Cardiogenic shock Severe hypotension (systolic BP < 70)	0.5 - 30 μg/min titrated to ffect To prepare infusion: Mix 4 mg in 250 ml (16 μg/ml). Titrate to desired effect.	• Relatively contraindicated in hypovolemic patients • Should not be administered in the same IV line as alkaline solutions • Use with caution in patients with ischemic heart disease as myocardial O_2 requirements may ↑ • Extravasation may result in tissue sloughing or necrosis

DRUG	MECHANISM OF ACTION/EFFECTS	INDICATIONS	DOSAGE	PRECAUTIONS
Dopamine **Trade Name:** Intropin, Dopastat **Class:** Sympathomimetic Natural catecholamine	Precursor of epinephrine that has dopaminergic, α and β-adrenergic receptor stimulating actions **Dose-related Effects:** **Low dose (1-2 μg/kg/min):** • Dilates renal and mesenteric vessels • May not $\uparrow$ heart rate or blood pressure at this dose range **2-10 μg/kg/min:** • Predominant β-adrenergic stimulating properties → $\uparrow$ force of contraction, minimal $\uparrow$ in heart rate → $\uparrow$ cardiac output **> 10 μg/kg/min:** • α effects dominate → renal, mesenteric, peripheral arterial and venous vasoconstriction → $\uparrow$ systemic vascular resistance and preload, $\uparrow$ heart rate $\uparrow$ BP **> 20 μg/kg/min:** • Effects similar to norepinephrine	Hypotension that occurs with symptomatic bradycardia Hypotension that occurs after return of spontaneous circulation Cardiogenic shock	Only administered by IV infusion, never as a bolus 5 - 20 μg/kg/min, titrated to desired effect **To mix infusion:** 400 mg dopamine in 250 ml (or 800 mg dopamine in 500 ml) → 1600 μg/ml concentration	• MAO inhibitors potentiate effects of dopamine • May induce tachycardia necessitating $\downarrow$ dosage or discontinuation of infusion • Extravasation may result in tissue sloughing or necrosis - monitor IV site closely • Should not be administered with alkaline solutions - inactivates dopamine • **Do not discontinue abruptly - taper gradually** • Should be infused via an infusion pump • Should be infused via a central vein - if central venous access not possible, use a large peripheral vein (antecubital vein) • **Correct hypovolemia before administration of dopamine**

5. Dopamine:

   1. may cause tissue sloughing or necrosis if extravasation occurs during administration
   2. is useful in the management of hypertension
   3. should not be administered simultaneously with sodium bicarbonate
   4. may produce a paradoxical intracellular acidosis

   a. 1, 3
   b. 2, 4
   c. 1, 2
   d. 3, 4

6. Calcium chloride is not indicated in the management of:

   a. hypocalcemia
   b. hyperkalemia
   c. pulseless electrical activity
   d. calcium channel blocker toxicity

7. The correct dose range for an epinephrine infusion is:

   a. 2-10 μg/min
   b. 10-30 μg/min
   c. 2-4 μg/kg/min
   d. 5-20 μg/kg/min

8. Morphine sulfate:

   a. increases anxiety
   b. decreases venous capacitance
   c. decreases myocardial oxygen demand
   d. increases systemic vascular resistance

9. Sodium bicarbonate administration is classified as a Class I (definitely helpful) intervention in which of the following circumstances?

   a. hypoxic lactic acidosis
   b. prolonged resuscitation efforts
   c. cyclic antidepressant overdose
   d. known preexisting hyperkalemia

10. The type of drug that inhibits the effects of epinephrine and norepinephrine released from sympathetic nerve endings is known as a(n):

    a. sympatholytic
    b. anticholinergic
    c. sympathomimetic
    d. parasympatholytic

11. The recommended lidocaine dose in VF is:

    a. 1-3 mg titrated to effect
    b. 0.5-1.0 mg/kg slow IV bolus
    c. 1-1.5 mg/kg repeated in 5-10 minutes for a maximum dose of 3 mg/kg
    d. 6 mg rapid IV bolus repeated if necessary in 1-2 minutes with 12 mg

12. Verapamil may be useful in which of the following situations?

    a. cerebral failure
    b. symptomatic third-degree AV block
    c. Wolff-Parkinson-White (WPW) syndrome
    d. narrow-complex paroxysmal supraventricular tachycardia

13. Isoproterenol:

    1. is a pure β-adrenergic stimulator
    2. slows conduction through the AV junction
    3. causes renal and mesenteric vasoconstriction at higher doses
    4. may be used as a temporary measure in the management of torsades de pointes

    a. 1, 2
    b. 2, 3
    c. 1, 4
    d. 3, 4

14. Adenosine:

    a. is a pure β-adrenergic stimulator
    b. is used to suppress ventricular ectopy
    c. increases systolic blood pressure and dilates the renal and mesenteric vasculature
    d. is a first-line agent in the management of stable paroxysmal supraventricular tachycardia

15. The recommended infusion rate for dobutamine is:

    a. 1-2 mg/min

    b. 2-4 mg/min

    c. 5-10 μg/min

    d. 2-20 μg/kg/min

16. An adrenergic drug:

    a. decreases cardiac contractility

    b. is a medication that decreases a bodily function or activity

    c. causes effects like those of the sympathetic division of the autonomic nervous system

    d. causes effects like opposite those of the sympathetic division of the autonomic nervous system

17. Propranolol, Atenolol and Metoprolol are examples of:

    a. β-adrenergic blockers

    b. α-adrenergic blockers

    c. calcium channel blockers

    d. β-adrenergic stimulating agents

18. Procainamide:

    a. may cause hypotension

    b. is useful in the treatment of AV blocks

    c. is useful in the management of torsades de pointes

    d. is a first-line agent in the management of narrow-QRS paroxysmal supraventricular tachycardia

19. The recommended dose for atropine administration via the endotracheal tube is:

    a. 1-1$^1/_2$ times the IV dose

    b. 2-2$^1/_2$ times the IV dose

    c. the same as the IV dose

    d. none of these - atropine should not be administered via this route

20. Dobutamine:

    a. stimulates β-1 receptors $\rightarrow$ increased myocardial contractility

    b. stimulates α-1 receptors $\rightarrow$ dilation of renal and mesenteric blood vessels

    c. stimulates α-1, β-1 and β-2 receptors $\rightarrow$ increased heart rate, AV conduction and myocardial contractility

    d. stimulates α-1 receptors $\rightarrow$ peripheral vasoconstriction and increased peripheral vascular resistance

21. A 50 year old female is complaining of chest pain, dizziness and nausea. Her blood pressure is 62/38, respirations 18. The cardiac monitor shows a sinus bradycardia at 48/minute with frequent, multi-formed PVCs. Your first choice of drug and dosage will be:

    a. sublingual nitroglycerin
    b. morphine 1-3 mg IV bolus
    c. atropine 0.5-1.0 mg IV bolus
    d. lidocaine I-1.5 mg/kg IV bolus

22. Which of the following are calcium channel blockers?

    a. atenolol, diltiazem
    b. diltiazem, verapamil
    c. verapamil, propranolol
    d. metoprolol, diltiazem, verapamil

23. Thrombolytic therapy:

    1. should be administered by the first physician competent in making the diagnosis of acute MI
    2. should be used in conjunction with aspirin therapy
    3. may lead to significant complications, including intracranial bleeding
    4. when indicated, should be administered as soon as possible after the onset of symptoms

    a. 1, 4
    b. 2, 3
    c. 1, 2, 4
    d. 1, 2, 3, 4

24. Atropine:

    a. stimulates beta receptors
    b. stimulates dopaminergic receptors
    c. blocks the sympathetic division of the autonomic nervous system
    d. blocks the parasympathetic division of the autonomic nervous system

25. The initial dose of bretylium for a patient in VT with a pulse is:

    a. 5-10 mg/kg IV rapid IV bolus
    b. 5 mg over 3-5 minutes IV bolus
    c. 1 mg/kg IV bolus over 3-5 minutes
    d. 5-10 mg/kg IV infusion over 8-10 minutes

26. Dopamine, when infused at a dose range of 2-10 μg/kg/min, will most likely produce which of the following effects?

    a. bronchodilation
    b. cerebral anoxia
    c. increased salivation
    d. increased inotropic effect

27. Lidocaine is not indicated in which of the following situations?

    a. VT with a pulse
    b. wide-complex tachycardia of uncertain origin
    c. prophylactic use in the setting of suspected acute MI
    d. VT/VF that persist after defibrillation and administration of epinephrine

28. Furosemide:

    1. is a β-adrenergic stimulator
    2. is indicated in the management of acute pulmonary edema
    3. is administered as an initial bolus of 5 mg/kg slow IV bolus over 1-2 minutes
    4. is a venodilator and potent diuretic

    a. 1, 2
    b. 2, 4
    c. 1, 3
    d. 3, 4

29. It is thought that a total dose of __ mg of atropine results in full vagal blockade in humans.

    a. 0.5 mg
    b. 1.0 mg
    c. 2.0 mg
    d. 3.0 mg

30. Stimulation of β-1 receptors results in:

    a. peripheral vasoconstriction
    b. dilation of renal and mesenteric blood vessels
    c. increased heart rate, increased force of myocardial contraction
    d. relaxation of vascular and bronchial smooth muscle

31. The recommended initial adult IV dose of epinephrine in VF is:

    a. 1 mg every 3-5 minutes
    b. 1 mg/kg every 3-5 minutes
    c. 5 mg/kg every 5-10 minutes
    d. 2-5 mg every 15-30 minutes

32. Sodium nitroprusside:

    a. is a potent, rapid-acting arterial and venous peripheral vasodilator
    b. is indicated in cases of severe hypotension (systolic blood pressure < 70 mm Hg)
    c. is a Class IIa recommendation (probably helpful) in cases of calcium channel blocker toxicity
    d. is the preferred vasodilator in acute myocardial infarction, especially when complicated by congestive heart failure

33. Bretylium tosylate is used in the management of:

    a. congestive heart failure
    b. VF refractory to lidocaine
    c. symptomatic first degree AV block
    d. narrow-QRS supraventricular tachycardia

34. Lidocaine:

    1. is metabolized in the liver
    2. is the drug of choice in the management of ventricular escape rhythms
    3. decreases the ventricular fibrillation threshold
    4. in therapeutic doses, has no significant effect on myocardial contractility

    a. 1, 4
    b. 2, 3
    c. 1, 3
    d. 2, 4

35. A 63 year old male is complaining of shortness of breath and chest pain. The cardiac monitor shows a sinus rhythm at 80 beats/minute with frequent, R on T PVCs occurring at a rate of 8-10/minute and runs of VT. A total of 2 mg/kg of lidocaine was administered in bolus doses and the ectopy appears to be resolved. At what rate should the continuous lidocaine drip be infused?

    a. 1 mg/minute
    b. 2 mg/minute
    c. 3 mg/minute
    d. 4 mg/minute

36. Which of the following may prolong the QT interval?

    a. morphine
    b. atropine
    c. epinephrine
    d. procainamide

37. Sodium bicarbonate:

    a. blocks the renal reabsorption of sodium
    b. is a first-line treatment for cardiac arrest
    c. should not be administered in the same IV line with catecholamines
    d. should be administered with an initial bolus of 1 mEq/kg, repeated thereafter with the same dose every 10 minutes

38. Diltiazem:

    1. is a first-line agent used in the management of cardiogenic shock
    2. may decrease myocardial contractility
    3. may be of benefit in the management of atrial fibrillation or atrial flutter with a rapid ventricular response
    4. is administered as an initial dose of 2.5-5.0 mg IV bolus over 2 minutes

    a. 1, 2
    b. 2, 3
    c. 1, 4
    d. 3, 4

39. Which of the following decrease myocardial oxygen requirements?

    a. atropine, morphine
    b. epinephrine, atropine
    c. nitroglycerin, morphine
    d. norepinephrine, nitroglycerin

40. Oxygen, preferably 100%, should be administered as soon as possible to all patients with cardiac or pulmonary arrest or other patient with suspected hypoxemia, regardless of cause.

    a. true
    b. false

41. Norepinephrine:

    a. is a ventricular antidysrhythmic
    b. is a first-line agent used in the management of chest pain
    c. is a potent vasodilator used in the management of severe hypertension
    d. is recommended in the management of severe hypotension (systolic BP < 70 mm Hg)

42. Which of the following is administered by intravenous bolus?

    a. atropine
    b. dopamine
    c. dobutamine
    d. isoproterenol

43. Which of the following statements regarding adenosine is INCORRECT?

    a. adenosine has an extremely short half-life
    b. adenosine should be administered at an IV site as proximal to the heart as possible
    c. side effects seen with adenosine administration are long lasting due to adenosine's potent effects on the arterial vasculature
    d. PSVT may recur after administration of adenosine and may necessitate a repeat bolus of the drug or use of another antidysrhythmic

44. Medications used in the management of the stable patient with a wide-QRS complex tachycardia of uncertain origin include:

    1. bretylium
    2. lidocaine
    3. adenosine
    4. verapamil

    a. 1, 2
    b. 1, 2, 3
    c. 2, 3, 4
    d. 1, 4

45. The recommended continuous infusion rate for bretylium is:

    a. 1-2 mg/min
    b. 1-4 mg/min
    c. 2-4 mg/min
    d. 2-10 μg/kg/min

46. Atropine:

    1. is useful in treating symptomatic sinus bradycardia
    2. depresses AV node and sinus node activity
    3. may worsen myocardial ischemia due to excessive increases in heart rate
    4. may be beneficial in symptomatic AV block at the nodal level

    a. 1, 2, 4
    b. 1, 3, 4
    c. 1, 2, 3
    d. 2, 3, 4

47. The primary side effect of nitroglycerin administration is:

    a. hypokalemia, due to excessive diuresis
    b. hypotension, which may worsen myocardial ischemia
    c. vasoconstriction, which may excessively elevate blood pressure
    d. prolongation of the QT interval, which may precipitate torsades de pointes

48. Magnesium sulfate, when administered in pulseless VT or VF, is administered at a dose of:

    a. 2.5-5.0 mg slow IV bolus
    b. 5 mg/kg IV bolus and repeated in 5 minutes with 10 mg/kg
    c. 1.5 mg/kg and repeated in 3-5 minutes with the same dose
    d. 1-2 grams diluted in 10 ml and administered IV over 1-2 minutes

49. Furosemide should be:

    a. administered rapid IV push
    b. administered slowly over one-two minutes
    c. mixed in 50 ml of D5W and infused over 8-10 minutes
    d. mixed in 250 ml of D5W and infused via an infusion pump over a 24 hour period

50. All of the following are endpoints of procainamide administration EXCEPT:

    a. hypertension develops
    b. the dysrhythmia is suppressed
    c. a total of 17 mg/kg has been administered
    d. the QRS widens by 50% of its original width

CARDIOVASCULAR PHARMACOLOGY ANSWER SHEET

1.	A	B	C	D	26.	A	B	C	D
2.	A	B	C	D	27.	A	B	C	D
3.	A	B	C	D	28.	A	B	C	D
4.	A	B	C	D	29.	A	B	C	D
5.	A	B	C	D	30.	A	B	C	D
6.	A	B	C	D	31.	A	B	C	D
7.	A	B	C	D	32.	A	B	C	D
8.	A	B	C	D	33.	A	B	C	D
9.	A	B	C	D	34.	A	B	C	D
10.	A	B	C	D	35.	A	B	C	D
11.	A	B	C	D	36.	A	B	C	D
12.	A	B	C	D	37.	A	B	C	D
13.	A	B	C	D	38.	A	B	C	D
14.	A	B	C	D	39.	A	B	C	D
15.	A	B	C	D	40.	A	B	C	D
16.	A	B	C	D	41.	A	B	C	D
17.	A	B	C	D	42.	A	B	C	D
18.	A	B	C	D	43.	A	B	C	D
19.	A	B	C	D	44.	A	B	C	D
20.	A	B	C	D	45.	A	B	C	D
21.	A	B	C	D	46.	A	B	C	D
22.	A	B	C	D	47.	A	B	C	D
23.	A	B	C	D	48.	A	B	C	D
24.	A	B	C	D	49.	A	B	C	D
25.	A	B	C	D	50.	A	B	C	D

CARDIOVASCULAR PHARMACOLOGY QUIZ ANSWERS

QUESTION	ANSWER	RATIONALE	JAMA PAGE REFERENCE
1	C	Assess the patient's breath sounds. If they are clear, administer a fluid challenge of normal saline or lactated Ringer's to rule out hypovolemia as a possible cause of his hypotension. If no improvement in the patient's blood pressure, administer dopamine.	2209
2	B	Digoxin ↓ heart rate (negative chronotrope) and ↑ force of contraction (positive inotrope).	2210
3	B	Amrinone is a third-line agent that may be useful in the management of severe CHF refractory to diuretics, vasodilators and conventional inotropic agents. Amrinone's effects are similar to those of dobutamine. This drug should be used in conjunction with hemodynamic monitoring. Administration may exacerbate myocardial ischemia and/or worsen ventricular ectopy.	2209
4	B	Bronchodilation and vasodilation are effects of β-2 receptor stimulation.	N/A
5	A	Dopamine may be of value in the management of hypotension that occurs with symptomatic brady-cardia, cardiogenic shock and in cases of hypoten-sion that occurs after return of spontaneous circulation. Dopamine administration may result in tissue sloughing or necrosis if extravasation occurs during administration. Administration of *sodium bicarbonate* may produce a paradoxical intracellu-lar acidosis.	2209
6	C	Calcium is indicated in cases of hyperkalemia, calcium channel blocker toxicity and hypocalcemia. It is not indicated in the management of pulseless electrical activity.	2209

7	A	If epinephrine is administered by continuous IV infusion, the infusion should begin at 1 μg/min and titrate upward to desired response (2-10 μg/min).	2209
8	C	Morphine ↑ venous capacitance (pools blood in the periphery), ↓ venous return (preload), ↓ systemic vascular resistance (afterload), ↓ *myocardial oxygen demand*, ↑ pain threshold	2206
9	D	Sodium bicarbonate is a Class I intervention in cases of known preexisting hyperkalemia. It is a Class IIa intervention in cyclic antidepressant overdose; Class IIb in prolonged resuscitation efforts and Class III in hypoxic lactic acidosis.	2217, 2219, 2220
10	A	A sympatholytic is a drug that *inhibits* the effects of epinephrine and norepinephrine released from sympathetic nerve endings.	N/A
11	C	In VF, lidocaine is administered as a 1-1.5 mg/kg IV bolus and repeated in 5-10 minutes for a maximum total dose of 3 mg/kg.	Updated since JAMA publication.
12	D	Verapamil is indicated in *narrow*-complex paroxysmal supraventricular tachycardia (with a normal or elevated blood pressure).	2207
13	C	Isoproterenol is a pure β-adrenergic stimulator that increases heart rate (+ chronotrope) and may be used as a temporary measure in the management of torsades de pointes. (Magnesium sulfate is the drug of choice). Dopamine causes renal and mesenteric vasoconstriction at higher doses.	2207
14	D	Adenosine is a first-line agent in the management of paroxysmal narrow-QRS supraventricular tachycardia.	2207
15	D	The recommended infusion rate for dobutamine is 2-20 μg/kg/min.	2209
16	C	An adrenergic drug causes effects like those of the sympathetic division of the autonomic nervous system.	N/A
17	A	Propranolol, atenolol and metoprolol are examples of β-adrenergic blockers.	2206

18	A	Procainamide administration may result in hypotension. This drug should be avoided in the management of torsades de pointes. Procainamide is a *third-line* agent in the management of *wide-complex* tachycardia of uncertain origin and PSVT. Procainamide is not indicated in the management of any type of AV block.	2206
19	B	Lidocaine, atropine and epinephrine are ACLS drugs that may be administered via the endotracheal tube. The recommended dose is $2-2^{1}/_{2}$ times the IV dose.	2205
20	A	Dobutamine stimulates β-1 receptors which $\uparrow$ myocardial contractility.	2209
21	C	Atropine is the drug of choice in bradycardia accompanied by hypotension, PVCs, chest pain or dyspnea. SL nitroglycerin and morphine should be withheld at this time due to the patient's significant hypotension.	2231
22	B	Diltiazem and verapamil are calcium channel blockers. Propranolol, atenolol and metoprolol are β-adrenergic blockers.	2207
23	D	Thrombolytic therapy, when indicated, should be administered as soon as possible after the onset of symptoms by the first physician competent in making the diagnosis of acute MI. Thrombolytics should be used in conjunction with aspirin and may lead to significant complications including systemic fibrinogen depletion, intracranial bleeding and systemic bleeding.	2181, 2211, 2230-2231
24	D	Atropine *blocks* the parasympathetic division of the autonomic nervous system.	2207
25	D	5-10 mg/kg of bretylium, when administered to the patient with a pulse, should be mixed in 50 ml of D5W and infused over 8-10 minutes to avoid the nausea and vomiting associated with more rapid infusion.	2206
26	D	When administered at a dose range of 2-10 μg/kg/min, dopamine will produce an $\uparrow$ inotropic effect.	2209

27	C	*Prophylactic* lidocaine administration is no longer recommended.	2206
28	B	Furosemide (lasix) is a venodilator and potent diuretic used in the management of acute pulmonary edema. The initial dose is usually 0.5-1.0 mg/kg slow IV bolus over 1-2 minutes.	2211
29	D	A total dose of 3 mg of atropine is believed to result in full vagal blockade in humans.	2207
30	C	Stimulation of β-1 receptors will result in an ↑ heart rate and ↑ force of myocardial contraction. Peripheral vasoconstriction is an α-1 effect. Dilation of renal and mesenteric blood vessels is a dopaminergic effect. Stimulation of β-2 receptors results in relaxation of vascular and bronchial smooth muscle.	N/A
31	A	The recommended initial adult IV dose of epinephrine in VF is 1 mg which may be repeated every 3-5 minutes. After the initial bolus, alternative dosing schedules may be used.	2208
32	A	Sodium nitroprusside is a potent, rapid-acting arterial and venous peripheral vasodilator used in the management of heart failure and hypertension. Norepinephrine is indicated in cases of severe hypotension (systolic BP <70 mm Hg). Calcium chloride is indicated in cases of calcium channel blocker toxicity. Nitroglycerin is the preferred vasodilator in acute myocardial infarction, especially when complicated by congestive heart failure.	2210
33	B	Bretylium tosylate is indicated in the management of pulseless VT/VF refractory to lidocaine.	2206
34	A	Lidocaine is a ventricular antidysrhythmic that is metabolized in the liver and is useful in the management of VF, VT, significant ventricular ectopy (R on T PVCs, runs of VT seen in the setting of acute MI/ischemia) and wide-complex tachycardia of uncertain origin. Lidocaine increases the ventricular fibrillation threshold and is contraindicated in ventricular escape rhythms.	2206

35	C	The lidocaine infusion should be administered at a dose of 1 mg/min more than the total mg/kg dose administered. Since 2 mg/kg was administered, the drip should be infused at a rate of 3 mg/minute.	N/A
36	D	Drugs that may prolong the QT interval include procainamide, disopyramide (Norpace), quinidine, some cyclic antidepressants, and organic pesticides, among others.	2206
37	C	Sodium bicarbonate inactivates simultaneously administered catecholamines. When sodium bicarbonate is administered, the initial dose is 1 mEq/kg followed by 1/2 this dose every 10 minutes thereafter.	2211
38	B	Diltiazem is a calcium channel blocker that is indicated in the management of multifocal atrial tachycardia, atrial fibrillation or atrial flutter with a rapid ventricular response. Diltiazem may result in decreased myocardial contractility and should be avoided in the patient with severe cardiac failure.	2207
39	C	Nitroglycerin and morphine ↓ myocardial oxygen requirements. Epinephrine, norepinephrine and atropine ↑ myocardial oxygen requirements.	2206
40	A	Oxygen, preferably 100%, should be administered as soon as possible to all patients with cardiac or pulmonary arrest or other patient with suspected hypoxemia, regardless of cause.	2205
41	D	Norepinephrine is a potent vasoconstrictor used in cases of severe hypotension (systolic BP < 70 mm Hg).	2209
42	A	Atropine is administered as an IV bolus medication.	2207
43	C	Side effects seen with adenosine administration (most commonly flushing, chest pain and dyspnea) are usually short-lived, resolving in 1-2 minutes, due to adenosine's extremely short half-life.	2207

44	B	Medications used in the management of wide-QRS tachycardia of uncertain origin include lidocaine, adenosine, procainamide and bretylium.	2223
45	A	The recommended continuous IV infusion rate for bretylium is 1-2 mg/min.	2206
46	B	Atropine is useful in treating symptomatic sinus bradycardia and may be beneficial in symptomatic AV block at the nodal level. Atropine increases the rate of discharge of the sinus node and improves AV conduction. Atropine should be used with caution in patients with acute myocardial ischemia or infarction because excessive increases in heart rate may worsen ischemia or increase the zone of infarction.	2207
47	B	The primary side effect of nitroglycerin administration is hypotension, which may worsen myocardial ischemia.	2210
48	D	In pulseless VT and VF, magnesium sulfate is administered at a dose of 1-2 grams diluted in 10 ml and administered IV over 1-2 minutes.	2208
49	B	Furosemide should be administered by IV bolus slowly over 1-2 minutes.	2211
50	A	Procainamide should be discontinued if hypotension develops, the dysrhythmia is suppressed, a total of 17 mg/kg has been administered or the QRS widens by 50% of its original width.	2206

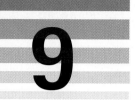

9 Intravenous Techniques

Objectives

Upon completion of this chapter, you will be able to:

1. Describe the indications for IV therapy.
2. Describe the advantages of peripheral venipuncture over central venous access.
3. Describe the advantages of central venous access over peripheral venipuncture.
4. Describe the indications for central venous access.
5. List four local complications common to all IV techniques.
6. List four systemic complications common to all IV techniques.
7. Identify anatomical landmarks for cannulation of the femoral, internal jugular and subclavian veins.
8. Describe the sites of first choice for cannulation if no IV is in place at the time of cardiac arrest.

Indications for IV Therapy

1. Administer drugs and fluids
2. Obtain venous blood
3. Insert catheters into the central circulation

Establishing an IV Lifeline

1. Routine part of advanced life support
2. As early as possible

TYPES OF IV CANNULAS

Hollow Needles

1. Indwelling plastic catheters inserted over a hollow needle
2. Indwelling plastic catheters inserted through a hollow needle or over a guide wire

Catheter-Over-The-Needle

1. After venipuncture, catheter introduced and needle removed
2. Length of catheter limited by length of needle
3. Puncture in vein exactly size of catheter which reduces possibility of bleeding around venipuncture site

Catheter-Through-The-Needle

1. Catheter pushed into vein through needle
2. Risk of sharp tip of needle shearing off the end of the catheter and producing a catheter-fragment embolus
   a. Never pull backward through the needle
   b. If you cannot advance the catheter through the needle, you must remove both the needle and catheter
3. Seldinger Technique with Guidewire
   a. Guidewire inserted into the vein through the needle and needle removed
   b. Catheter inserted over the guidewire into the vein and the guidewire removed
   c. Use of guidewire eliminates the hazard of catheter-fragment embolus
   d. If cannot pass guidewire through needle:
      - Remove guidewire and reattach syringe
      - Reposition needle in the vein
      - Remove the syringe and reinsert the guidewire
4. Introducer sheath may be inserted over guidewire; introducer and guidewire removed leaving sheath in place through which a large catheter can be passed

SELECTION OF CATHETERS

Plastic catheter

14-16 gauge in adult

Some advocate 18 gauge maximum if thrombolytic therapy is a consideration

Length depends on site of insertion

PRINCIPLES COMMON TO ALL IV TECHNIQUES

1. Peripheral or central venous access preferable to intracardiac injection during CPR

2. If an internal jugular or subclavian IV line is in place when an arrest occurs, it should be used for drug administration during the resuscitation effort.

3. If no IV exists prior to the arrest, sites of first choice are the antecubital or external jugular veins.

4. If spontaneous circulation does not return after initial drug administration via a peripheral vein, a central line can be placed

5. Even one unsuccessful central line attempt is a strong relative contraindication to initiation of thrombolytic therapy

6. Distal wrist and hand veins and saphenous veins in the legs are the least favorable sites for drug administration in cardiac arrest since blood flow from the distal extremities is markedly diminished.

7. Femoral veins are best avoided unless a long cannula can be passed above the level of the diaphragm

8. Strict aseptic technique may not be possible

9. Preferred solution in cardiac arrest = normal saline or lactated Ringer's solution

COMPLICATIONS COMMON TO ALL IV TECHNIQUES

Local Complications

Hematoma formation

Cellulitis

Thrombosis

Phlebitis

Systemic Complications

Sepsis

Pulmonary thromboembolism

Catheter-fragment embolism

Air embolism

PERIPHERAL VENIPUNCTURE

Advantages

1. Effective route for drugs during CPR
2. Does not require interruption of CPR
3. Easier to learn than central venous access
4. Results in fewer complications
5. Preferred sites in cardiac arrest = antecubital veins or external jugular
6. IV drugs should be administered rapidly by bolus injection during CPR and followed with a 20 ml bolus of IV fluid and elevation of the extremity

Disadvantages

1. In circulatory collapse, vein may be absent
2. Phlebitis common with saphenous vein
3. Should be used only for administration of isotonic solutions; hypertonic or irritating solutions may cause pain and phlebitis
4. When administered via a peripheral vein, drugs require 1-2 minutes to reach the central circulation

PERIPHERAL VENIPUNCTURE - EXTERNAL JUGULAR VEIN

Anatomy

1. Lies superficially along the lateral portion of the neck
2. Extends from the angle of the mandible and passes downward until it enters the thorax at a point just above the middle of the clavicle and ends in the subclavian vein

Advantages

1. Usually easy to cannulate
2. Is considered a peripheral vein
3. Provides rapid access to the central circulation

Disadvantages

1. May not be readily accessible during an arrest situation due to rescuers working to manage the airway
2. IV may be easily dislodged and positional with head movement

CENTRAL VENOUS ACCESS

Indications

1. Emergency access to venous circulation
2. Central venous pressure measurement
3. Administration of hypertonic or irritating solutions
4. Passing catheters into the heart and pulmonary circulation

CENTRAL VENOUS ACCESS - FEMORAL VEIN

Anatomy

1. The femoral vein lies directly medial to the femoral artery
2. If a line is drawn between the anterior superior iliac spine and the symphysis pubis, the femoral artery runs directly across the midpoint - medial to that point is the femoral vein
3. If the femoral artery pulse is palpable, the artery can be located with a finger and the femoral vein will lie immediately medial to the pulsation. A finger should remain on the artery to ease landmark identification and to avoid insertion of the catheter into the artery.

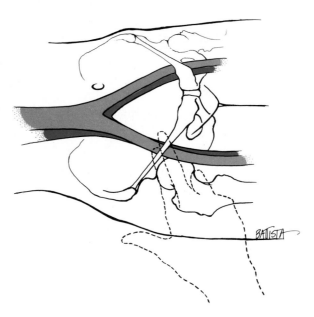

Figure 9-1   Anatomy of the femoral vein.

Femoral Vein - Advantages

1. Does not interrupt CPR
2. Vein does not collapse like peripheral veins
3. Once cannulated, there is easy access to the central circulation

Femoral Vein -
Disadvantages

1. If pulse absent, vein may be hard to locate
   - During CPR, the femoral vein pulsates and is easier to palpate than the femoral artery since arterial flow is low
2. Long delivery time of drugs into the central circulation unless a long line that extends above the diaphragm is used (due to decreased flow to the extremities)
3. Complication rate may be higher, especially involving thrombosis and infection, than for peripheral veins

Femoral Vein -
Complications

1. Thrombosis or phlebitis may extend to the deep or iliac veins or vena cava
2. Arterial cannulation may result in loss of limb
3. Hematoma

CENTRAL VENOUS ACCESS
INTERNAL JUGULAR VENIPUNCTURE

Anatomy

Runs from the base of the skull downward along the carotid artery until it enters the chest to meet with the subclavian vein behind the clavicle

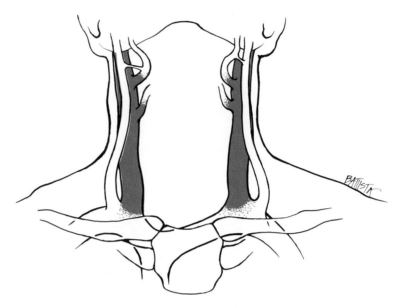

Figure 9-2   Anatomy of the internal jugular vein.

Internal Jugular - Specific Principles

Right side of neck preferred

- Dome of the right lung and pleura are lower than the left
- More or less a straight line to the right atrium
- Thoracic duct not in the way (empties on the LEFT side)

Internal Jugular - Advantages

1. Less risk of pneumothorax with this technique vs subclavian
2. Hematomas in the neck are visible and more easily compressible
3. Easier access during CPR than subclavian
4. Rapid access to central circulation possible even if peripheral veins are collapsed

Internal Jugular - Disadvantages

1. Adjacent structures easily damaged
2. More training required than peripheral venipuncture
3. May interrupt CPR
4. Higher complication rate than with peripheral venipuncture
5. Higher complications with thrombolytic therapy
6. Limits patient neck movement

CENTRAL VENOUS ACCESS
SUBCLAVIAN VENIPUNCTURE

Anatomy

1. Approximately 3-4 cm long and 1-2 cm in diameter
2. Is a continuation of the axillary vein, beginning at the point where this vein crosses over the first rib and under the medial half of the clavicle
3. The subclavian vein is immobilized by small attachments to the first rib and clavicle
4. The subclavian merges with the internal jugular vein to form the innominate (brachiocephalic) vein

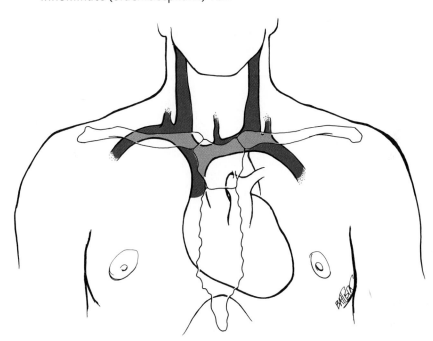

Figure 9-3   Anatomy of the subclavian vein.

Subclavian - Advantages

More subsequent patient neck movement with prolonged cannulation

Subclavian - Disadvantages

1. Significant risk of pneumothorax, hemothorax, subclavian artery puncture
2. More training required than peripheral venipuncture
3. May interrupt CPR
4. Higher complication rate than with peripheral venipuncture
5. Higher complications with thrombolytic therapy

INTERNAL JUGULAR AND SUBCLAVIAN VENIPUNCTURE – SPECIFIC COMPLICATIONS

Local Complications

1. Hematoma may compromise airway
2. Damage to adjacent artery, nerve or lymphatic duct
3. Perforation of endotracheal tube cuff

Systemic Complications

1. Pneumothorax - need follow-up on chest roentgenogram
2. Hemothorax
3. Air embolism
4. Infiltration into mediastinum or pleural space
5. Dysrhythmias from catheter tip

Special
Resuscitation
Situations **10**

Objectives

Upon completion of this chapter, you will be able to:

1. Identify at least four situations not initially involving the heart that may cause cardiac arrest.
2. Define ischemic and hemorrhagic stroke.
3. List five signs/symptoms of a stroke.
4. Describe the emergency management of a stroke.
5. Define hypothermia.
6. Describe the signs and symptoms associated with mild, moderate and severe hypothermia.
7. Describe the recommended basic and advanced life support measures in the management of the severely hypothermic patient.
8. Define drowning, near-drowning, immersion syndrome and secondary drowning.
9. Describe the recommended basic and advanced life support measures in the management of the near-drowning victim.
10. List four possible causes of traumatic cardiac arrest.
11. Describe the prehospital and hospital management of traumatic cardiac arrest.
12. Describe the management of the victim of electrocution and lightning strike.
13. Define supine hypotension.
14. Describe the management of the pregnant cardiac arrest victim.

Special Resuscitation
Situations

1. Stroke
2. Hypothermia
3. Near-Drowning
4. Trauma
5. Electrical Shock/Lightning Strike
6. Pregnancy

STROKE

Definition

An illness of sudden onset caused by occlusion or rupture of a blood vessel in the brain

Cerebral Blood Flow

80% of blood flow to the brain is supplied by the carotid arteries
20% is supplied through the vertebrobasilar system

Etiology

Ischemic stroke

- Accounts for approximately 75% of strokes
- An artery is blocked by a blood clot that either developed within the vessel (thrombosis) or arose from another source (such as the heart) and travelled to the brain (embolism)

Hemorrhagic stroke

- Result of a ruptured cerebral blood vessel
- Bleeding can occur adjacent to the brain (subarachnoid hemorrhage) or
- Bleeding can occur into the substance of the brain (intracerebral hemorrhage)

Warning Signs

Transient ischemic attack (TIA)

- Most important forecaster of ischemic stroke
- Reversible episode of focal neurological dysfunction lasting < 24 hours

Signs/Symptoms

- Can occur alone but are most common in combination
- Can be most severe at the beginning, wax and wane or progressively worsen
- Clinical presentations of ischemic and hemorrhagic stroke overlap
- Loss of consciousness may be transient with resolution by the time the patient is seen by medical personnel
- Patients with subarachnoid hemorrhage may have an intense headache without focal neurological signs
- Headaches, disturbances in consciousness, nausea and vomiting more prominent with intracranial hemorrhages

Clinical Presentation	• Alteration in consciousness (coma, stupor, seizures, delirium)
	• Intense or unusually severe headache of sudden onset or any headache associated with a decreased level of consciousness or neurological deficit; unusual and severe neck of facial pain
	• Aphasia (incoherent speech or difficulty understanding speech)
	• Facial weakness or asymmetry (paralysis of the facial muscles, usually noted when the patient speaks or smiles); may be on the same side or opposite side from limb paralysis
	• Incoordination, weakness, paralysis, or sensory loss of one or more limbs; usually involves one half of the body, particularly the hand
	• Ataxia (poor balance, clumsiness or difficulty walking)
	• Visual loss; may be a partial loss of visual field
	• Dysarthria (slurred or indistinct speech)
	• Intense vertigo, double vision, unilateral hearing loss, nausea, vomiting, photophobia or phonophobia
Physical Exam - Airway and Ventilation	• Airway obstruction may be a problem if the patient is comatose
	• Inadequate ventilation or aspiration may result in hypoxia and hypercarbia and exacerbate stroke
	• Must ensure adequate airway, intubate as necessary
Physical Exam - Vital Signs	• Check vital signs frequently and note changes
	• Abnormal respirations particularly prominent in comatose patients
	• Hypertension may indicate:
	• underlying hypertension
	• stress reaction to the event
	• physiological response to decreased brain perfusion
	• Blood pressure often returns to normal without treatment
	• Cardiac dysrhythmias
	• may be underlying cardiac cause of brain embolism
	• may be consequence of brain injury
	• life-threatening dysrhythmias are an important early complication of stroke, particularly of intracranial hemorrhage

Physical Exam - Neuro Assessment	Level of consciousness (LOC) most important

Physical Exam - Neuro Assessment

Level of consciousness (LOC) most important
- Decreased LOC is indicative of major brain injury and identifies those stroke patients most at risk of dying
- Glasgow Coma Scale used to assess severity of neuro deficit (assesses eye opening, motor and verbal responses)
- Pupillary responses
- Spontaneous limb movement
- Meningeal signs (rigidity of the neck)

Diagnosis of Stroke

Important to differentiate ischemia vs hemorrhagic stroke because prognosis and treatment markedly different

Emergency Treatment

IV Therapy
- NS or LR at 30 ml/hr
- Unless the patient is hypotensive, rapid infusions should be avoided due to risk of increased intracranial pressure
- Avoid D5W unless hypoglycemia STRONGLY suspected (is hypotonic and may increase cerebral edema)

Antihypertensive drugs
- Use rarely and cautiously in ischemic stroke
- Lower BP to estimated prestroke levels in hemorrhagic stroke

Anticonvulsants
- Phenytoin (15 mg/kg orally or IV no faster than 50 mg/min if administered IV)
- Diazepam (10 mg IV)
- Phenobarbital (15 mg/kg IV) - use caution for respiratory depression

Treatment of increased intracranial pressure
- Fluid restriction
- Elevate head of bed
- Intubation and hyperventilation to a PCO2 of 25-28 mm Hg (an effective, although temporary, measure when the patient is developing signs of herniation)
- Control of agitation and pain
- Mannitol 1-2 g/kg IV over 5-10 min
- Dexamethasone value unproven in patients with stroke
- Heparin value unproven - should not be administered to a patient who has had a stroke until CT has eliminated the possibility of intracranial bleeding
- Use of thrombolytics is currently being researched
- Neuro consult

HYPOTHERMIA

Definition	Accidental fall in core temperature < 35° C
	Severe accidental hypothermia = body temperature < 30° C (86° F)
	May "appear clinically dead due to marked depression of brain and cardiovascular function, but full resuscitation with intact neuro recovery is possible, although unusual
	Peripheral pulses and respiratory efforts may be difficult to detect, but life-saving procedures should not be withheld based on clinical presentation"[1]
Incidence	Very young/very old among those most susceptible
May be missed if thermometer won't read below 34.4° C
	Major areas of heat loss from the body are the head and the back of the neck
Common Clinical Situations	1. Immersion in cold water
2. Cold weather exposure
3. Impaired thermogenesis - elderly, infants, drug or alcohol ingestion, diabetes, infection
Commonly Associated Conditions	1. Alcohol or other drug ingestion
2. Diabetes (especially hypoglycemia)
3. Endocrine disorders
4. Near-drowning
5. Trauma (especially head injury)
6. Sepsis
Physiological Conditions	1. Inhibits release of ADH - diuresis/dehydration
2. Hematocrit and viscosity of blood increased
3. Insulin release and peripheral utilization inhibited and may result in an elevated blood sugar
Mild Hypothermia (34-36° C)	Shivering
Early rise in blood pressure and respiratory rates
Lack of coordination
Memory loss
Poor judgment
Pale, cold, dry skin

Pulmonary Edema	Occurs in 75% of cases
	Seawater shifts intravascular fluid into alveoli
	Freshwater injures capillary membrane and removes surfactant

Associated Injuries

- Spinal cord injury (diving)
- Air embolism or the "bends" (SCUBA)
- Hypothermia

Possible Underlying Causes

- Alcohol or other drug ingestion
- Hypoglycemia
- Seizures
- Suicide, homicide or child abuse

Rescue Breathing

- Rescue breathing with mouth-to-mouth technique should be started as soon as the victim's airway can be opened and protected and the rescuer's safety can be assured (usually when the victim is in shallow water or out of the water)
- Suspect neck injury in diving accidents
  - support neck in NEUTRAL position
  - chin-lift or jaw-thrust WITHOUT head tilt
  - float victim on a back support before being removed from the water
- There is no need to clear the airway of aspirated water, however, debris, gastric contents or other foreign material may need to be removed
- Bag-mask ventilation, intubation

"An attempt to remove water from the breathing passages by any means other than suction is usually unnecessary and apt to be dangerous because it may eject gastric contents and cause aspiration."[2]

Heimlich Maneuver

- Delays initiation of ventilation and breathing
- Should be used ONLY if rescuer suspects foreign matter is obstructing the victim's airway or if the victim does not respond appropriately to mouth-to-mouth ventilation

Chest Compressions

- Should not be attempted in the water unless the rescuer has had special training in in-water CPR
- Pulse may be difficult to palpate because of peripheral vasoconstriction and decreased cardiac output
- After removal from the water, if a pulse cannot be felt, initiate CPR at once

Advanced Cardiac Life Support	100% oxygen
	Suction PRN
	Cardiac monitor
	(Orogastric tube)
	Warming if hypothermic

"Every submersion victim, even one who requires only minimal resuscitation and regains consciousness at the scene, should be transferred to a medical facility for follow-up care."[3]

Prognosis — Survival possible with prolonged immersion in cold water - especially in children

TRAUMATIC CARDIAC ARREST

Possible Causes

1. Severe central neurological injury with secondary cardiovascular collapse
2. Hypoxia secondary to respiratory arrest resulting from neurological injury, airway obstruction, large open pneumothorax, or severe tracheo-bronchial laceration or crush
3. Direct and severe injury to vital structures (heart, aorta)
4. Underlying medical problems that led to the injury (such as sudden VF)
5. Severely diminished oxygen delivery
6. Injuries in a cold nvironment (eg, fractured leg) complicated by secondary severe hypothermia

Prehospital - Cardiac Arrest with Injuries

1. Rapid extrication
2. Nasotracheal intubation ONLY if patient breathing
3. Orotracheal intubation with in-line stabilization of the neck by an assistant
4. IV line placement enroute to trauma center
5. Needle decompression if tension pneumothorax present

Hospital - Cardiac Arrest with Injuries

1. If VF, defibrillate
2. Secure airway with endotracheal tube (if not already done) or surgical airway if needed
3. Suspect tension pneumothorax, if present, needle decompression
4. Volume resuscitation
5. Emergency thoracotomy
   - permits open chest CPR, control of thoracic and extrathoracic hemorrhage, aortic cross-clamping, pericardiocentesis

ELECTROCUTION/LIGHTNING STRIKE

Factors Determining
the Impact of Electrical
Injury[4]

1. Amperage
   - 1 ampere is approximately equal to the amount of current passing through a 100-watt lightbulb.[5]
2. Voltage
   - Low-voltage = 1000 volts or less
   - High-voltage = more than 1000 volts
3. Resistance of tissues
   - Nerves = least resistance
   - Muscle and blood vessels have decreased resistance
   - Fat and bone have increased resistance
   - Moisture decreases skin resistance
4. Type of current
   - Alternating current (household and industrial current) is 3 times more damaging than direct current because of its ability to:
     - Cause tetanic muscle contractions
     - "Freeze" the victim to the circuit
5. Pathway of current
   - Hand-to-hand (transthoracic) pathway more likely to be fatal than hand-to-foot (vertical) or foot-to-foot (straddle)
6. Duration of current
   - The longer the contact with source, the greater the body exposure to current, the greater the damage

Current Intensity →
Effects

< 1 mA   tingling

5-30 mA   "let go current"

40-50 mA   respiratory arrest

> 100 mA   ventricular fibrillation

> 10 A   prolonged apnea

Thermal Injury

1. Electricity travels along nerves and blood vessels
2. Burns may be superficial or deep; may extend to bone

Secondary Injury	1. Fractures
	• Cervical spine
	• Skull (due to fall, blunt trauma)
	• Femur
	• Humerus
	2. Closed head injury
	3. Peripheral nerve injury
	4. Myoglobinuria
	• Myoglobin is a protein released as a result of muscle damage
	• Increased myoglobin levels may lead to kidney failure
	• Increase IV fluids to prevent renal shutdown
Cardiac and Respiratory Arrest	1. Primary cause of death due to electrical injury
	2. VF or ventricular asystole may occur as a direct result of electric shock
	• VF most commonly occurs with low-voltage shocks
	• Asystole most commonly occurs with high-voltage shocks
	3. Respiratory arrest may occur secondary to:
	• Electric current passing through the brain and causing inhibition of medullary respiratory center function
	• Tetanic contraction of the diaphragm and chest wall musculature during current exposure
	• Prolonged paralysis of respiratory muscles which may continue for minutes after the electric shock has terminated
Electric Shock - Basic Life Support	The prognosis for recovery from electric shock is not readily predictable because the amperage and duration of the charge are usually unknown.
	1. Assure rescuer safety
	2. Turn off current
	3. ABCs of CPR
	4. Protect cervical spine and treat injuries

Electric Shock -
Advanced Cardiac
Life Support

VF, ventricular asystole and other serious dysrhythmias should be treated per the ACLS guidelines for these rhythms

- Intubation may be difficult in patients with electrical burns of the face, mouth or anterior neck due to soft-tissue swelling
- If hypovolemic shock or significant tissue destruction, rapid IV fluid administration is indicated to:
  - Counteract shock
  - Correct ongoing fluid losses
  - Maintain a diuresis to avoid renal shutdown due to myoglobinuria
- Early consult with surgical/burn specialist

Lightning Injury

1. Lightning acts as massive DC countershock and depolarizes the entire myocardium at once resulting in asystole
2. Death in 30% of victims
3. Primary cause of death in lightning-strike victims is cardiac arrest due to VF or ventricular asystole
4. If multiple victims struck, treat those who are unconscious first

PREGNANCY

Cardiovascular Changes
in Mother

1. Maternal blood volume and cardiac output increased up to 50%
2. Maternal heart rate, minute volume and oxygen consumption increased
3. Pulmonary functional residual capacity, systemic and pulmonary vascular resistance decreased
4. Uterine blood flow increases from 2 (normal) to 20% of cardiac output

Precipitants of Cardiac
Arrest

Pulmonary embolism

Trauma

Peripartum hemorrhage with hypovolemia

Amniotic fluid embolism

Congenital and acquired cardiac disease

Congestive heart failure, MI

Supine Hypotension

- Supine position compresses aorta and inferior vena cava → decreased venous return → decreased cardiac output
- Rolling mother to left side (left lateral recumbent position) may increase cardiac output by 25%

Cardiac Arrest

If VF is present, it should be treated with defibrillation according to the VF algorithm

CPR

Airway management

Displace uterus to the left

Pharmacologic therapy WITHOUT any modifications

- Vasopressors such as epinephrine, norepinephrine and dopamine should NOT be withheld when clinically indicated

Volume replacement

If there is potential fetal viability, prompt cesarean section should be considered if the above measures have failed to restore effective circulation.

Decision to perform cesarean should be made rapidly (within 4-5 minutes of the arrest) to maximize chances of maternal and infant survival

REFERENCES

1. Emergency Cardiac Care Committee and Subcommittees, American Heart Association. Guidelines for cardiopulmonary resuscitation and emergency cardiac care, *JAMA* 268:2244, 1992.

2. Emergency Cardiac Care Committee and Subcommittees, American Heart Association. Guidelines for cardiopulmonary resuscitation and emergency cardiac care, *JAMA* 268:2246, 1992.

3. Emergency Cardiac Care Committee and Subcommittees, American Heart Association. Guidelines for cardiopulmonary resuscitation and emergency cardiac care, *JAMA* 268:2246, 1992.

4. Cooper MA. Electrical and lightning injuries. *Emerg Med Clin N Am* 2:489, 1984.

5. Langley RL, Dunn KA, Esinhart JD. Lightning fatalities in North Carolina, 1972-1988. *NC J Med* 52:281, 1991.

6. Cooper MA. Electrical injury. In: Callaham ML, ed. *Current Therapy in Emergency Medicine.* Philadelphia: BD Decker; 928, 1987.

INTRAVENOUS TECHNIQUES/SPECIAL RESUSCITATION SITUATIONS QUIZ

1. Which of the following is NOT an advantage of internal jugular vein cannulation over subclavian vein cannulation?

    a. less risk of pleural puncture
    b. easier to cannulate during CPR
    c. allows more free movement for the patient
    d. hematomas are visible and easily compressible

2. The most important forecaster of ischemic stroke is:

    a. the patient's age
    b. history of diabetes
    c. a transient ischemic attack (TIA)
    d. history of cardiovascular disease

3. Supine-hypotension:

    a. occurs as a result of prolonged labor
    b. occurs as a result of significant spinal injury
    c. is characterized by a tearing sensation in the abdomen and constant pain
    d. occurs as a result of compression of the abdominal aorta and inferior vena cava by the gravid uterus when the mother is supine

4. Where is the femoral vein relative to the femoral artery?

    a. medial
    b. lateral
    c. anterior
    d. posterior

5. Sudden death triggered by vagally induced dysrhythmias after cold water immersion best defines:

    a. drowning
    b. near-drowning
    c. immersion syndrome
    d. secondary drowning

6. An 83 year old female was found by a neighbor in her apartment. It is early December and prehospital personnel report there was no heat in her apartment. The patient is conscious, although slow to respond to your questions. She is pale and cold to the touch. The patient states she is on a limited income and could not afford the cost of heating her apartment. Her blood pressure is 80/60, respirations are 18 per minute. The cardiac monitor shows a sinus rhythm at 64 beats/minute. A thermometer has recorded her temperature as 34°C (93°F). Initial management of this patient should include:

    a. initiate CPR, defibrillate with 200, 300, 360J

    b. administer warm, humidified oxygen; establish an IV of normal saline and administer 6 mg of adenosine rapid IV bolus

    c. administer warm, humidified oxygen; establish an IV of normal saline and apply warm packs to the neck, axilla and groin

    d. administer warm, humidified oxygen; establish an IV of 5% dextrose in water and administer epinephrine 1 mg IV bolus

7. Signs and symptoms associated with a cerebrovascular accident may include all of the following EXCEPT:

    a. dehydration and weight loss

    b. facial weakness or asymmetry

    c. altered level of consciousness

    d. difficulty with speech or vision

8. Which of the following statements regarding central venous access is INCORRECT?

    a. if a femoral pulse is absent, the vein may be difficult to locate

    b. central venous lines may be successfully placed, even when peripheral perfusion is poor

    c. central venous access technique requires more training than does peripheral venipuncture technique

    d. current ACLS guidelines recommend accessing the central circulation through an internal jugular site or infraclavicular subclavian site

9. The three components measured with the Glasgow Coma Scale are:

    a. eye opening, verbal response and motor response

    b. vital signs, eye opening and decorticate posturing

    c. level of consciousness, vital signs and respiratory pattern

    d. decorticate and decerebrate posturing and level of consciousness

10. A 38 year old female is in labor. She becomes suddenly short of breath, markedly diaphoretic and complains of a sharp pain in her chest. Your cardiac monitor shows a sinus tachycardia at 138/minute. You suspect this patient may be experiencing:

    a. uterine rupture
    b. a pulmonary embolism
    c. a myocardial infarction
    d. acute congestive heart failure

11. Local complications common to all intravenous techniques include:

    a. sepsis
    b. phlebitis
    c. air embolism
    d. catheter-fragment embolism

12. A transient ischemic attack usually lasts:

    a. 30-60 seconds
    b. 30 minutes to 1 hour
    c. no more than four hours
    d. several minutes or up to 24 hours

13. The greatest amount of heat is lost from the:

    a. head and feet
    b. feet and torso
    c. head and back of the neck
    d. upper and lower extremities

14. Which of the following statements regarding IV therapy during cardiac arrest is INCORRECT?

    a. a large-bore catheter should be used
    b. drugs administered during cardiac arrest should be administered by IV bolus
    c. drug delivery to the central circulation may be improved by administration of a 20 ml bolus of IV fluid and elevation of the extremity
    d. drugs administered by means of peripheral veins take four to five minutes to reach the central circulation

15. Intubation with hyperventilation when a patient is developing signs of herniation is an effective, although temporary, measure of lowering increased intracranial pressure.

    a. true
    b. false

16. Which of the following statements regarding emergency treatment of the patient suffering a stroke is INCORRECT?

    a. elevation of the head of the bed may help to lower increased intracranial pressure

    b. 5% dextrose in water is hypertonic and may decrease cerebral edema

    c. the IV solution(s) of choice are normal saline and lactated Ringer's solution

    d. unless the patient is hypotensive, rapid infusions should be avoided due to the risk of increasing cerebral edema

17. Which of the following correctly lists signs and symptoms of mild hypothermia (34-36° C)?

    a. rigidity, ventricular fibrillation, apnea

    b. loss of dexterity, tachycardia, hypertension, memory loss

    c. shivering, bradycardia, hypotension, altered level of consciousness

    d. hypotension, bradycardia, rigidity, altered level of consciousness

18. Leg veins are generally avoided for IV therapy due to:

    a. discomfort

    b. inadequate flow rates

    c. increased likelihood and severity of venous thrombosis

    d. increased likelihood of extravasation due to motion and downward position

19. Select the INCORRECT statement regarding near-drowning.

    a. when resuscitating the victim of a diving accident, neck injury should be suspected and the neck supported in a neutral position

    b. pulmonary edema may occur as a complication of near-drowning in both fresh and salt water

    c. hypoxemia is the most important major physiologic consequence of near-drowning

    d. the Heimlich maneuver should be employed as soon as possible to clear the airway of any aspirated water

20. Management of the unconscious, severely hypothermic patient with vital signs should include:

    1. gentle handling and cardiac monitoring
    2. initiation of CPR, withholding of IV medications and limiting shocks for VF/VT to a maximum of three
    3. endotracheal intubation to provide effective ventilation and reduce the risk of aspiration
    4. administration of warm, humidified oxygen and warm intravenous fluids

    a. 1, 2
    b. 2, 3
    c. 1, 2, 3
    d. 1, 3, 4

IV TECHNIQUES/SPECIAL RESUSCITATION SITUATIONS QUIZ ANSWER SHEET

1.   A   B   C   D

2.   A   B   C   D

3.   A   B   C   D

4.   A   B   C   D

5.   A   B   C   D

6.   A   B   C   D

7.   A   B   C   D

8.   A   B   C   D

9.   A   B   C   D

10. A   B   C   D

11. A   B   C   D

12. A   B   C   D

13. A   B   C   D

14. A   B   C   D

15. A   B   C   D

16. A   B   C   D

17. A   B   C   D

18. A   B   C   D

19. A   B   C   D

20. A   B   C   D

IV TECHNIQUES/SPECIAL RESUSCITATION SITUATIONS QUIZ ANSWERS

QUESTION	ANSWER	RATIONALE	JAMA PAGE REFERENCE
1	C	Cannulation of the internal jugular vein does not allow more free movement for the patient.	N/A
2	C	The most important forecaster of ischemic stroke is a transient ischemic attack (TIA).	2242
3	D	Supine hypotension occurs as a result of compression of the abdominal aorta and inferior vena cava by the gravid uterus when the mother is supine.	2249
4	A	The femoral vein is medial to the femoral artery.	N/A
5	C	Immersion syndrome is defined as delayed sudden death triggered by vagally induced dysrhythmias after cold water immersion.	N/A
6	C	Administer warm, humidified oxygen; establish an IV of normal saline and apply warm packs to the neck, axilla and groin.	2244-2245
7	A	Signs and symptoms of a cerebrovascular accident do not include dehydration or weight loss.	2242
8	D	Current ACLS guidelines recommend accessing the central circulation through an internal jugular site or **SUPRA**clavicular subclavian site. These sites/approaches should require less interruption of chest compressions than the INFRAclavicular approach.	2205
9	A	The three areas evaluated with the Glasgow Coma Scale are eye opening, best motor response and best verbal response.	N/A
10	B	This patient is most likely experiencing a pulmonary embolism.	N/A

11	B	Local complications include phlebitis, cellulitis, hematoma formation and thrombosis. Systemic complications include air embolism, sepsis, pulmonary thromboembolism and catheter-fragment embolism.	N/A
12	D	A transient ischemic attack may last for several minutes or hours but resolves within 24 hours.	2242
13	C	The greatest amount of heat is lost from the head and the back of the neck.	N/A
14	D	Drugs administered via peripheral veins take approximately 1-2 minutes to reach the central circulation.	2205
15	A	True. Intubation with hyperventilation when a patient is developing signs of herniation is an effective, although temporary, measure of lowering increased intracranial pressure.	2244
16	B	5% dextrose in water is **hypotonic** and may **increase** cerebral edema.	2243
17	B	Signs and symptoms of mild hypothermia include shivering, loss of dexterity, tachycardia, hypertension, hyperventilation, memory loss and poor judgment.	N/A
18	C	Leg veins are generally avoided because blood flow from the distal extremities is markedly diminished → ↑ likelihood and severity of venous thrombosis.	N/A
19	D	The Heimlich maneuver should be employed **ONLY** if you suspect foreign matter is obstructing the airway or if the victim does not respond appropriately to mouth-to-mouth ventilation (lack of chest rise, unable to ventilate).	2246
20	D	Initiation of CPR, withholding of IV medications and limiting shocks for VF/VT to a maximum of three are treatment measures used in the management of the severely hypothermic patient **without** vital signs.	2245

Putting It All Together

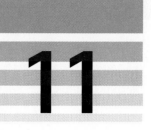

11

Objectives

Upon completion of this chapter, you will be able to:

1. Describe the role of each member of the resuscitation team.
2. Discuss the "phase response" of code organization.
3. Describe the principles of cardiac arrest management.
4. Discuss the AHA guidelines for management of:
   - VF/pulseless VT
   - Asystole
   - Pulseless electrical activity
   - Sustained VT with a pulse
     - Stable patient
     - Unstable patient
   - Polymorphic VT
   - PSVT (stable and unstable patient)
   - Atrial fibrillation and flutter with a rapid ventricular response
   - Symptomatic bradycardia
5. Identify the immediate goals of postresuscitation care.
6. Describe four complications of resuscitation.
7. Describe the management of types of organ failure.
8. Describe common signs of distress.
9 Define and describe burnout.
10. Identify three reasons why it may be difficult for the health care professional to convey the news of a sudden death to family members.
11. Discuss the AHA protocol for conveying news of a sudden death to family members.
12. Discuss the AHA recommendations for Critical Incident Debriefing.

Goals of the Resuscitation Team

1. Reestablish spontaneous circulation and respiration
2. Preserve function in vital organs during resuscitation

Team Leader -
Responsibilities

1. Broad skills of organization and performance

2. Supervision and direction of team members
   - Determines when to start and stop CPR
   - Assures that pulses are assessed when appropriate
   - Reviews the adequacy of ventilation and ensures that airway adjuncts are used properly
   - Evaluates hand position for CPR, depth of cardiac compressions, proper rate and sequence of CPR
   - Assures that interruptions for intubation, defibrillation or moving the patient do not exceed 30 seconds
   - Responsible for the safety of all members of the resuscitation team - especially when procedures such as defibrillation are performed

3. Patient assessment
   - Patient's history
   - Resuscitation status
   - Physical findings
   - Cardiac rhythm
   - Problem-solving
   - Recognizing and determining the cause of equipment malfunction
   - Determining the cause of abnormal laboratory results
   - Reasons for unsuccessful therapy
     - Endotracheal tube placement
     - Assessment of breath sounds
     - Pulses with CPR
     - Correct paddle position

CODE ORGANIZATION - "PHASE RESPONSE"

Phase I - Anticipation

Rescuers either move to the scene of a possible cardiac arrest or await the arrival of a possible cardiac arrest from outside the hospital. Steps necessary are:
- Analyze prehospital data
- Gather the resuscitation team
- State leadership
- Delineate duties
- Prepare and check equipment
- Position oneself

Phase II - Entry

The team leader introduces him/herself and begins to obtain data to initiate the resuscitation effort:
- Obtain entry vital signs
- Perform early transfer
- Gather concise history
- Repeat vital signs

Phase III - Resuscitation

The team leader directs the resuscitation team through the various protocols.

The team LEADER should:
- Communicate his/her observations
- Actively seek suggestions from team members

Team MEMBERS should:
- State vital signs every 5 minutes or with any change in the monitored parameters
- State when procedures and medications are completed
- Request clarification of any orders
- Provide primary and secondary assessment information

Phase IV - Maintenance

Vital signs have stabilized. The team should stabilize and secure the patient and repeatedly reevaluate the ABCs.

Vulnerable Period!

Phase V - Family Notification

"Telling the living" must be done with "honesty, sensitivity, and promptness"

Phase VI - Transfer

Patient care is transferred to a team "of equal or greater expertise"

Phase VII - Critique   Every resuscitation effort should be critiqued by the team. This provides:

- Avenue to express grieving
- Opportunity for education
- Feedback to hospital and prehospital personnel

ACLS TEAM MEMBERS

Primary Roles

1. Airway Management including:
   - ventilation, oxygenation, intubation, suctioning
2. External chest compressions
3. Use of "quick-look" paddles and defibrillator
4. Establishment of IV access and administration of drugs
5. Placement of ECG electrodes
6. Operation of the ECG machine
7. Patient assessment
8. Cardiac rhythm analysis
9. Communication with base hospital (if prehospital personnel)

Support Roles

1. Management of supplies
2. Assistance with procedures
3. Documentation of the resuscitation effort
4. Liaison functions
5. Crowd control

PRINCIPLES OF CARDIAC ARREST MANAGEMENT

Upon recognition of arrest

Initiate CPR and call for help

Arrival of resuscitation team, emergency cart, monitor, defibrillator

1. Equipment
   - Cardiac board
   - Oropharyngeal airway
   - Mouth-to-mask or bag-valve-mask with oxygen tubing
   - Oxygen supply and regulator
2. Intervention
   - Place patient on cardiac board
   - Ventilate with 100% oxygen with oropharyngeal airway and mask
   - Continue chest compressions

Identification of team leader	1. Assesses patient 2. Directs and supervises team members 3. Solves problems 4. Obtains history and information leading to arrest situation
Rhythm diagnosis	• Use quick-look paddles if leads are not already attached • Connect limb leads
Prompt defibrillation if indicated	Use correct algorithm Resume CPR
Intubation	• Connect suction equipment • Intubate patient in < 30 seconds • Confirm tube position (assess breath sounds, chest rise) • Hyperventilate and oxygenate
Venous access	Large-bore catheter IV solution:normal saline or lactated Ringer's Peripheral: antecubital or external jugular vein
Drug administration	Use correct algorithm
Ongoing assessment of response to therapy	• Assess pulses with CPR • Assess adequacy of ventilation • Assess pulses after interventions and/or rhythm change • Assess breathing with return of pulse • Assess blood pressure, if pulse present • Consider decision to terminate efforts if no response
Documentation	Accurately record the events during the resuscitation effort
Drawing arterial and venous blood	Treat as needed based on results
Controlling or limiting crowd	Dismiss those not required

TREATMENT PRIORITIES

• Rapid defibrillation for VF or pulseless VT
• Effective CPR
• Secure airway (preferably with endotracheal intubation) and the administration of 100% oxygen
• Epinephrine to maintain coronary and brain perfusion

USING ALGORITHMS

- General guidelines
- A change in the rhythm or a change in the pulse changes the algorithm
- Continually reassess → conditions change

VENTRICULAR FIBRILLATION
PULSELESS VENTRICULAR TACHYCARDIA

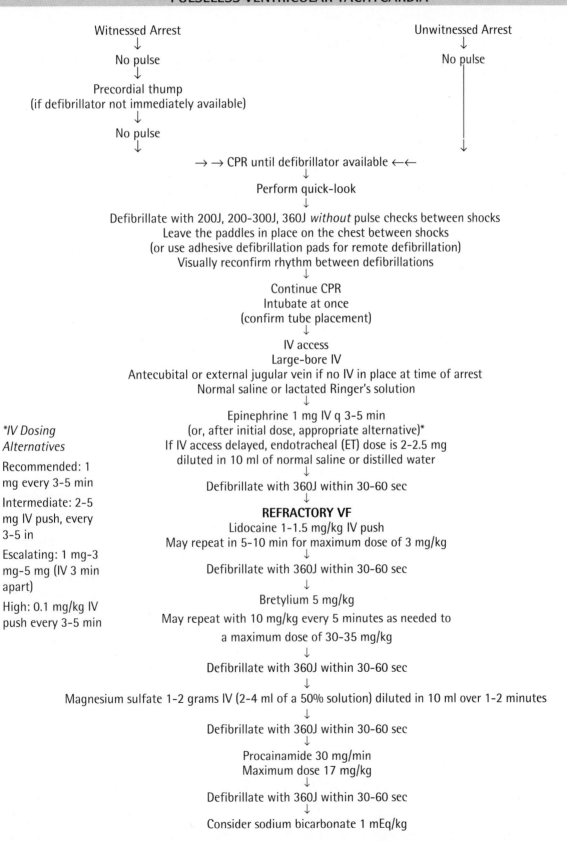

Witnessed Arrest   Unwitnessed Arrest
↓   ↓
No pulse   No pulse
↓
Precordial thump
(if defibrillator not immediately available)
↓
No pulse
↓

→ → CPR until defibrillator available ←←
↓
Perform quick-look
↓
Defibrillate with 200J, 200-300J, 360J *without* pulse checks between shocks
Leave the paddles in place on the chest between shocks
(or use adhesive defibrillation pads for remote defibrillation)
Visually reconfirm rhythm between defibrillations
↓
Continue CPR
Intubate at once
(confirm tube placement)
↓
IV access
Large-bore IV
Antecubital or external jugular vein if no IV in place at time of arrest
Normal saline or lactated Ringer's solution
↓
Epinephrine 1 mg IV q 3-5 min
(or, after initial dose, appropriate alternative)*
If IV access delayed, endotracheal (ET) dose is 2-2.5 mg
diluted in 10 ml of normal saline or distilled water
↓
Defibrillate with 360J within 30-60 sec
↓
REFRACTORY VF
Lidocaine 1-1.5 mg/kg IV push
May repeat in 5-10 min for maximum dose of 3 mg/kg
↓
Defibrillate with 360J within 30-60 sec
↓
Bretylium 5 mg/kg
May repeat with 10 mg/kg every 5 minutes as needed to
a maximum dose of 30-35 mg/kg
↓
Defibrillate with 360J within 30-60 sec
↓
Magnesium sulfate 1-2 grams IV (2-4 ml of a 50% solution) diluted in 10 ml over 1-2 minutes
↓
Defibrillate with 360J within 30-60 sec
↓
Procainamide 30 mg/min
Maximum dose 17 mg/kg
↓
Defibrillate with 360J within 30-60 sec
↓
Consider sodium bicarbonate 1 mEq/kg

*IV Dosing
Alternatives

Recommended: 1
mg every 3-5 min

Intermediate: 2-5
mg IV push, every
3-5 in

Escalating: 1 mg-3
mg-5 mg (IV 3 min
apart)

High: 0.1 mg/kg IV
push every 3-5 min

ASYSTOLE

CPR
↓
Intubate
(Confirm tube placement)
Assess breath sounds
Observe chest rise
↓
Establish IV access
Large bore IV
Normal saline or lactated Ringer's
Antecubital or external jugular
↓
Confirm rhythm in another lead
Change lead-selector on the monitor
If using paddles in quick-look mode, rotate paddles 90°
↓
Consider possible causes:
H(x4)AD

Hypoxia
Hypokalemia
Hyperkalemia
Hypothermia
Acidosis (preexisting)
Drug overdose
↓
Consider immediate transcutaneous pacing
↓
Epinephrine 1 mg IV every 3-5 minutes
(or, after initial dose, appropriate alternative*)
ET dose 2-2.5 mg diluted in 10 ml of normal saline or distilled water
↓
Atropine 1 mg IV every 3-5 minutes to maximum 3 mg
ET dose 2-2.5 mg diluted in 10 ml of normal saline or distilled water
↓
Consider sodium bicarbonate 1 mEq/kg
↓
Consider termination of efforts
↓
IV Dosing Alternatives
Recommended: 1 mg every 3-5 min
Intermediate: 2-5 mg IV push, every 3-5 in
Escalating: 1 mg-3 mg-5 mg (IV 3 min apart)
High: 0.1 mg/kg IV push every 3-5 min

PULSELESS ELECTRICAL ACTIVITY

CPR
↓

Intubate (confirm tube placement)
Assess breath sounds
Observe chest rise
↓

Establish IV access
Large bore IV
Normal saline or lactated Ringer's
Antecubital or external jugular
500 ml fluid challenge
↓

Assess blood flow using Doppler
↓

Consider underlying causes
↓

MATCH(x4)ED
Myocardial Infarction (massive acute)
Acidosis (severe)
Tension pneumothorax
Peri**C**ardial tamponade
Hypoxia (severe)
Hypothermia
Hypovolemia
Hyperkalemia
Pulmonary **E**mbolism (massive)
Drug overdose
↓

Epinephrine 1 mg IV every 3-5 minutes
(or, after initial dose, appropriate alternative*)
ET dose 2-2.5 mg diluted in 10 ml of normal saline or distilled water
↓

Atropine 1 mg IV every 3-5 minutes to maximum 3 mg
ET dose 2-2.5 mg diluted in 10 ml of normal saline or distilled water
↓

Consider sodium bicarbonate 1 mEq/kg

*IV Dosing Alternatives

Recommended: 1 mg
every 3-5 min

Intermediate: 2-5 mg IV
push, every 3-5 min

Escalating: 1 mg-3 mg-
5 mg IV 3 min apart

High: 0.1 mg/kg IV push
every 3-5 min

Sodium Bicarbonate use:
Class I (definitely helpful) if known preexisting hyperkalemia
Class IIa (Probably helpful)
- If known preexisting bicarbonate-responsive acidosis
- If overdose with cyclic antidepressants
- To alkalinize the urine in drug overdoses
Class IIb (Possibly helpful)
- If intubated and long arrest interval
- Upon return of spontaneous circulation after long arrest interval
Class III (Not indicated, may be harmful)
- Hypoxic lactic acidosis

SYMPTOMATIC BRADYCARDIA

Symptomatic narrow-
QRS bradycardia
• Sinus bradycardia
• Junctional rhythm
• Second-degree AV block,
type I
• Third-degree (narrow QRS)

Signs/symptoms:
Chest pain
Shortness of breath
Decreased level of con-
sciousness
Shock
 Pulmonary congestion
CHF
Acute MI

ABCs, O_2, IV
↓
Atropine 0.5–1.0 mg IV every 3–5 minutes
to maximum 2–3 mg
↓
Transcutaneous pacemaker
↓
Dopamine infusion 5–20 μg/kg/min
↓
Epinephrine infusion 2–10 μg/min
↓
Isoproterenol infusion (low dose)

Symptomatic wide-QRS AV
block bradycardia
• Second-degree AV block,
type II
• Third degree (wide-QRS)

ABCs, O_2, IV
↓
Transcutaneous pacemaker
(prepare for transvenous pacemaker)
↓
Dopamine infusion 5–20 μg/kg/min
↓
Epinephrine infusion 2–10 μg/min

ATRIAL FIBRILLATION/ATRIAL FLUTTER WITH A RAPID VENTRICULAR RESPONSE

Stable Patient

ABCs, O_2, IV
↓
Consider:

Diltiazem
0.25 mg/kg (20 mg) IV over 2 min followed 15 minutes
later with 0.35 mg/kg (25 mg) IV over 2 minutes
↓
β-blockers
Atenolol: 5-10 mg IV over 5 min
Esmolol: 500 μg/kg over 1 minute (loading dose) followed by
a maintenance infusion at 50 μg/kg/min over 4 minutes
Metoprolol: 5-10 mg slow IV push at 5 min intervals to total of 15 mg
Propranolol: Total dose of 0.1 mg/kg slow IV push divided into 3
equal doses at 2-3 in intervals
↓
Verapamil
2.5-5.0 mg slow IV bolus over 2 minutes
If no response, may repeat with 5-10 mg every
15-30 minutes to a maximum of 20 mg
↓
Digoxin
Procainamide
Quinidine
Anticoagulants

Unstable Patient

ABCs, O_2, IV
↓
Consider medications
↓
If the patient displays serious signs and symptoms,
prepare for immediate countershock
↓
Administer sedation whenever possible
↓

Atrial Flutter
Synchronized countershock with 50J, 100J, 200J, 300J, 360J

Atrial Fibrillation
Synchronized countershock with 100J, 200J, 300J, 360J

NARROW-QRS TACHYCARDIA (PSVT)

Stable Patient

ABCs, O$_2$, IV
↓
Vagal maneuvers
↓
Adenosine 6 mg *rapid* IV bolus
Consider decreasing the dose in patients on dipyridamole (Persantine)
Consider increasing the dose in patients on theophylline
↓
If needed, after 1-2 minutes:
Adenosine 12 mg rapid IV bolus
↓
If needed, after 1-2 minutes
Adenosine 12 mg rapid IV bolus
↓
Verapamil 2.5-5.0 mg slow IV bolus
↓
If needed, after 15-30 minutes:
Verapamil 5-10 mg slow IV bolus
↓
Consider Digoxin, β-blockers,
Diltiazem

Unstable Patient

ABCs, O$_2$, IV
↓
Consider medications
↓
If the patient displays serious signs and symptoms,
prepare for immediate countershock
↓
Administer sedation whenever possible
↓
Synchronized countershock
50, 100J, 200J, 300J, 360J

WIDE-COMPLEX TACHYCARDIA OF UNCERTAIN ORIGIN

Stable Patient

ABCs, O$_2$, IV
↓
Lidocaine 1–1.5 mg/kg
Repeat with 0.5–0.75 mg/kg every 5–10 minutes as needed
to a maximum of 3 mg/kg
↓
Adenosine 6 mg rapid IV bolus
Consider decreasing the dose in patients on dipyridamole (Persantine)
Consider increasing the dose in patients on theophylline
↓
If needed, in 1–2 minutes:
Adenosine 12 mg rapid IV bolus
↓
If needed, in 1–2 minutes:
Adenosine 12 mg rapid IV bolus
↓
Procainamide 20–30 mg/min
Maximum dose 17 mg/kg
(approximately 1.2 grams in a 70 kg patient)
↓
Bretylium 5–10 mg/kg *infusion*
in 50 ml D5W over 8–10 min
Maximum 30 mg/kg over 24 hours
↓
Consider synchronized countershock

Caution: Administration of verapamil may be lethal unless the wide-complex
tachycardia is known WITH CERTAINTY to be supraventricular in origin[1]

Unstable Patient

ABCs, O$_2$, IV
↓
Consider medications
↓
If the patient displays serious signs and symptoms,
prepare for immediate countershock
↓
Administer sedation whenever possible
↓
Synchronized countershock with
100J, 200J, 300J, 360J

NOTE: If undue delay in synchronization, or if clinical conditions are critical,
UNSYNC (defibrillate) at same energy.

SUSTAINED VENTRICULAR TACHYCARDIA WITH A PULSE

Stable Patient

ABCs, O$_2$, IV
↓
Lidocaine 1-1.5 mg/kg
Repeat with 0.5-0.75 mg/kg every 5-10 minutes as needed
to a maximum of 3 mg/kg
↓
Procainamide 20-30 mg/min to a maximum
dose of 17 mg/kg
↓
Bretylium 5-10 mg/kg *infusion* over
8-10 minutes
↓
Synchronized countershock with
100J, 200J, 300J, 360J

Unstable Patient

Signs/Symptoms:
- Dyspnea
- Chest pain
- Ischemia
- Infarction
- Hypotension
- Pulmonary edema, congestive heart failure
- Decreased level of consciousness

ABCs, O$_2$, IV
↓
Consider medications
↓
If the patient displays serious signs and symptoms,
prepare for immediate countershock
↓
Administer sedation whenever possible
↓
Synchronized countershock with
100J, 200J, 300J, 360J

If VF occurs during the course of synchronization:
- check pulse, check rhythm
- turn off the synchronizer switch
- defibrillate

NOTE: If undue delay in synchronization, or if clinical conditions are critical,
UNSYNC (defibrillate) at same energy.

Pulseless VT

Pulseless, apneic

Treat using VF algorithm → Defibrillate with 200J, 200-300J, 360J

POLYMORPHIC VENTRICULAR TACHYCARDIA

Stable Patient

1. Treatment of choice is transcutaneous ("overdrive") pacing
2. Drug therapy
   - Magnesium sulfate drug of choice (1-2 g IV over 1-2 min followed by same amount infused over 1 hour)
   - Isoproterenol 2-10 μg/min infusion

Unstable Patient
(sustained rhythm)

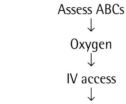

Assess ABCs
↓
Oxygen
↓
IV access
↓
Administer sedation whenever possible
↓
Unsynchronized countershock (defibrillation) with 200J, 200-300J, 360J

IMMEDIATE POSTRESUSCITATION CARE

- Reassess ABCs
- Continue airway support and 100% oxygen
- If hypotensive, administer dopamine infusion
- Begin infusion of lidocaine or bretylium (whichever was effective in converting rhythm)
  - Lidocaine contraindicated in ventricular escape rhythms
- Identify and correct underlying abnormalities
  - Chest roentgenogram
  - Lab work
  - 12-lead ECG

POSTRESUSCITATION CARE

Immediate Goals of
Postresuscitation Care

1. Provide cardiorespiratory support to optimize tissue perfusion - especially to the brain

2. Transport the patient to the hospital emergency department and then to an appropriately equipped critical care unit

3. Attempt to identify the precipitating cause of the arrest

4. Initiate measures such as antidysrhythmic therapy to prevent recurrence

Complications of
Resuscitation

Rib fractures
Pneumothorax
Hemopneumothorax
Pericardial tamponade
Intra-abdominal trauma
Misplaced endotracheal tube

OPTIMAL RESPONSE TO RESUSCITATION

Awake, responsive, spontaneously breathing patient

1. Apply ECG leads
2. Administer supplemental oxygen
3. If not already done, start IV infusion of normal saline
4. Change IV lines that were placed without proper sterile technique
5. If arrest rhythm was VF or VT and no antidysrhythmic was given:
   - Administer a lidocaine bolus
   - Follow with a continuous infusion
   - *CONTRAINDICATED in patients with ventricular escape rhythms*
6. If an antidysrhythmic was used successfully during the resuscitation effort, continue a maintenance infusion of that medication
7. Consider the precipitating cause of the arrest
   - Infarction
   - Electrolyte disturbances
   - Primary dysrhythmias
8. Consider thrombolytic therapy for:
   - Patients surviving resuscitations of short duration and minimial trauma
   - Evidence of acute MI on postresuscitation 12-lead ECG and with no contraindications
9. Exclude infarction in all patients
   - Serial ECGs and enzyme levels
10. Assess hemodynamic status, vital signs and urine output
11. Order:
    - 12-lead ECG
    - Portable chest roentgenogram
    - Arterial blood gas (ABG)
      - In candidates for thrombolytic therapy, draw ABGs only if less invasive assessment of oxygenation (pulse oximetry), ventilation (expired CO2) and acid-base status (venous sample) are unavailable
    - Electrolytes, glucose, creatinine, serum urea nitrogen, magnesium and calcium levels
      - Treat potassium, magnesium, calcium and sodium abnormalities aggressively
12. Transfer to special care unit for continuous care
    - Transfer with oxygen and ECG monitoring
    - Transfer with resuscitation equipment and trained personnel to accompany patient

SINGLE OR MULTIPLE ORGAN SYSTEM FAILURE

Patient Presentation

- Usually unconscious with endotracheal tube in place
- May or may not be spontaneously breathing
- May be unstable with respect to:
  - Cardiac rhythm
  - Cardiac rate
  - Blood pressure
  - Organ perfusion
- May be in a coma or show decreased responsiveness

Avoid hypoxemia and hypotension (exacerbates brain injury)

In most cases, acidemia of arrest spontaneously improves with adequate ventilation and reperfusion

Transfer to CCU

1. Maintain oxygenation and mechanical ventilation

2. Continue ECG monitoring

3. During transport, assess circulatory status with physical palpation of carotid or femoral pulses, continuous intra-arterial pressure monitoring or pulse oximetry

4. Transport patient with all necessary equipment and trained personnel able to perform immediate defibrillation and drug therapy if needed

Respiratory System

1. Perform complete examination and review chest roentgenogram
   - Pay special attention to complications of resuscitation
     - Pneumothorax
     - Improper endotracheal tube placement
     - Rib fractures
     - Hemopneumothorax
     - Pericardial tamponade
2. Provide ventilatory support
   - Level of mechanical support determined by:
     - Blood gas levels
     - Respiratory rate
     - Perceived work of breathing
   - The need for mechanical support decreases as spontaneous ventilations become more efficient
   - If high O_2 concentrations needed, determine if cause is pulmonary or cardiac dysfunction
     - If pulmonary problem, administration of O_2 using positive end-expiratory pressure (PEEP) may be indicated if the patient is stable
     - If cardiac problem, support failing myocardium
   - Adjust oxygen and ventilation therapy based on sequential ABGs, pulse oximetry and capnography results
   - Before extubation, evaluate pulmonary mechanics

Cardiovascular System

1. Perform complete physical examination
2. Evaluate vital signs and urine output
3. Compare 12-lead ECG with previous tracings (if available)
4. Evaluate:
   - Chest roentgenogram
   - Serum electrolyte levels (including calcium and magnesium)
   - Cardiac enzyme and isoenzyme levels
     - Enzyme levels may be elevated as a result of the resuscitation effort alone
5. If patient unstable, assess circulating fluid volume and ventricular function
   - Even mild hypotension can impair recovery of cerebral function
   - Intra-arterial blood pressure assessment
     - Permits better titration of catecholamine infusions
     - Remains accurate in patients with decreased cardiac output and vasoconstriction
6. In the critically ill patient, hemodynamic monitoring is usually required

Renal System

1. Perform urinary catheterization
   - Measure hourly urine output
   - Assess intake and output
     - Output includes:
       - Urine
       - Gastric secretions
       - Diarrheal fluid
       - Vomitus
2. In the oliguric patient, differentiation of prerenal failure vs acute renal failure may be assisted by:
   - Measurement of pulmonary occlusive pressure and cardiac output
   - Electrolyte values
   - Fractional excretion of filtered sodium
   - Urine sediment
3. Furosemide may maintain urine output despite developing renal failure
4. May need to use dopamine at low doses (1-3 μg/kg/min)
5. Use caution when administering nephrotoxic drugs or drugs eliminated by means of the kidneys
6. Consider dialysis with progressive renal failure

Central Nervous System

- Absence of circulation for 10 seconds results in decreased O_2 to brain and produces unconsciousness
- After 2-4 minutes, glucose and oxygen stores depleted
- After 4-5 minutes, ATP exhausted
- After extended hypoxemia or hypercarbia (or both), cerebral blood flow becomes dependent on cerebral perfusion pressure since autoregulation of cerebral blood flow is lost
  - Cerebral perfusion pressure = mean arterial pressure - intracranial pressure

If the patient is unresponsive, optimize cerebral perfusion pressure by:
- Maintaining normal or slightly elevated mean arterial pressure
- Reduce intracranial pressure if increased
  - Maintain normothermia and control seizure activity with phenobarbital, phenytoin or diazepam because hyperthermia and seizures increase brain oxygen requirements
  - Elevate the head of the bed to approximately 30° (promotes cerebral venous drainage)
  - Use care when performing tracheal suctioning
    - Increases intracranial pressure
    - Preoxygenate with 100% O_2 to help prevent hypoxemia

Gastrointestinal System	1. Insert nasogastric tube if bowel sounds are absent
	2. Increased incidence of stress ulceration and GI bleeding postresuscitation
	• Administer prophylactic antacid, H_2-blockers or sucralfate

PSYCHOLOGICAL FEATURES OF RESUSCITATION

Impact of Providing Help	Facing stress decreases anxiety levels
	Avoidance or distraction increases anxiety levels
	1. Unsuccessful CPR attempt may result in psychological dysfunction in volunteer emergency personnel
	• Vivid, involuntary, uncontrollable thoughts, feelings or mental images concerning the resuscitation effort
	2. Emergency personnel find "routine CPR" relatively unstressful
	• Major coping strategy is focusing on the patient (not on the bystanders, such as relatives)
	3. Deaths of young people and accidents involving major trauma most difficult

Signs of Distress	Nightmares
	Involuntary daytime recollections
	Anxiety
	Ruminations

DEATH, GRIEVING AND FAMILIES

Conveying News to the Family	1. Initial contact with the family will have a significant impact on the grief response
	• Inappropriate, incomplete or uncaring manner in the delivery of bad news may have a long-lasting psychological effect
	2. May be difficult for the health care professional
	• Physicians and other health care workers may not receive proper training as to how to convey death of a patient to the family
	• May be difficult to switch from "no time for feelings" during the resuscitation effort to the emotional postresuscitation situation
	• Feelings of failure and inadequacy may make it difficult to initially support and counsel the patient's family
	• Physician may feel isolated and second-guess decisions

PROTOCOL FOR CONVEYING NEWS OF A SUDDEN DEATH TO FAMILY MEMBERS[2]

Call the family if they have not been notified. Explain that their love one has been admitted to the emergency department and that the situation is serious. Survivors should not be told of the death over the telephone.

Obtain as much information as possible about the patient and the circumstances surrounding the death. Carefully go over the events as they happened in the emergency department.

Ask someone to take family members to a private area. Walk in, introduce yourself, and sit down. Address the closest relative.

Briefly describe the circumstances leading to the death. Go over the sequences of events in the emergency department. Avoid euphemisms such as "he's passed on," "she's no longer with us," or "he's left us." Instead, use the words "death," "dying," or "dead."

Allow time for the shock to be absorbed. Make eye contact, touch, and share. Convey your feelings with a phrase such as "You have my (our) sincere sympathy" rather than "I (we) are sorry."

Allow as much time as necessary for questions and discussion. Go over the events several times to make sure everything is understood and to facilitate further questions.

Allow the family the opportunity to see their relative. If equipment is still connected, let the family know.

Know in advance what happens next and who will sign the death certificate. Physicians may impose burdens on staff and family if they fail to understand policies about death certification and disposition of the body. Know the answers to these questions before meeting with the family.

Enlist the aid of a social worker or the clergy if not already present.

Offer to contact the patient's attending or family physician and to be available if there are further questions. Arrange for follow-up and continued support during the grieving period.

HELPING THE HELPERS

Stress Response

Chronic anxiety

Reactive depression

Burnout

- Results from cumulative stress in a work-related environment
- Leads to:
  - Job dissatisfaction
  - Poor job performance
  - Less enjoyment of life in general
- Can affect anyone
  - Those in helping professions particularly vulnerable
- Need to distinguish from major depression and posttraumatic stress disorder

Critical Incident Debriefing

1. Should occur after any situation in which workers are exposed to significant stress
2. Purpose:
   - Discussion of thoughts, feelings and performance
   - Expression of anxiety, guilt, anger and other emotions
   - "Grief work" facilitated and resolution accomplished
   - Allows review of critical responsibility
   - Provides continuing education or "practice reflections"

RECOMMENDATIONS FOR CRITICAL INCIDENT DEBRIEFING[3]

The debriefing should occur as soon as possible after the event, with all team members present.

Call the group together, preferably in the resuscitation room. State that you want to have a "code debriefing."

Review the events and conduct of the code. Include the contributory pathophysiology leading to the code, the decision tree followed, and any variations.

Analyze the things that were done wrong and especially the things that were done right. Allow free discussion.

Ask for recommendations for future resuscitative attempts.

All team members should share their feelings, anxieties, anger and possible guilt.

Team members unable to attend the debriefing should be informed of the process followed, the discussion generated, and the recommendations made.

The team leader should encourage team members to contact him or her if questions arise later.

REFERENCES

1. Emergency Cardiac Care Committee and Subcommittees, American Heart Association. Guidelines for cardiopulmonary resuscitation and emergency cardiac care, *JAMA* 268:2225, 1992.

2. Emergency Cardiac Care Committee and Subcommittees, American Heart Association. Guidelines for cardiopulmonary resuscitation and emergency cardiac care, *JAMA* 268:2233, 1992.

3. Emergency Cardiac Care Committee and Subcommittees, American Heart Association. Guidelines for cardiopulmonary resuscitation and emergency cardiac care, *JAMA* 268:2234, 1992.

Post-Test

1. Which of the following is considered a peripheral vein?

   a. femoral
   b. subclavian
   c. internal jugular
   d. external jugular

2. In the presence of acute myocardial damage or severe ischemia, susceptibility to dysrhythmias is greatest during the __ of symptom onset.

   a. first two weeks
   b. first three days
   c. first 4-6 minutes
   d. first several hours

3. The most common cause of pulseless electrical activity is:

   a. hypovolemia
   b. tension pneumothorax
   c. pericardial tamponade
   d. massive pulmonary embolism

4. Lidocaine may be lethal if administered for which of the following rhythms?

   a. ventricular tachycardia
   b. ventricular escape rhythm
   c. wide complex tachycardia of uncertain origin
   d. sinus tachycardia with frequent runs of ventricular tachycardia

5. Synchronized countershock is indicated for the unstable patient with all of the following rhythms EXCEPT:

   a. polymorphic ventricular tachycardia
   b. paroxysmal supraventricular tachycardia
   c. atrial flutter with a rapid ventricular response
   d. atrial fibrillation with a rapid ventricular response

A 58 year old male suffered a syncopal episode on the golf course. His friends have brought him to your Emergency Department for evaluation. The patient is awake, alert and oriented complaining of nausea and weakness. His blood pressure is 78/40, respiratory rate 14. The patient denies chest pain or shortness of breath although he is pale and diaphoretic. Breath sounds are clear and equal bilaterally. The patient has no significant past medical history although he states this is the third episode of "passing out" he has experienced in the past three months. The cardiac monitor displays the following rhythm:

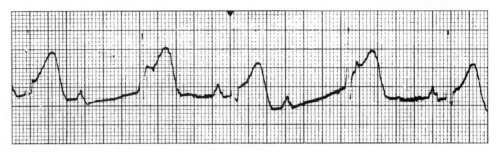

Figure 12-1

6. The rhythm displayed above is:

    a. second-degree AV block, type I

    b. second-degree AV block, type II

    c. complete (third-degree) AV block

    d. sinus bradycardia with a first degree AV block

7. Management of this patient would include:

    a. O_2, IV, morphine 1-3 mg IV, lidocaine 1-1.5 mg/kg IV bolus

    b. O_2, IV, vagal maneuvers, adenosine 6 mg rapid IV bolus

    c. O_2, IV, administer sedation, synchronized countershock with 100J

    d. O_2, IV, atropine 0.5-1.0 mg every 3-5 minutes as needed to a maximum of 2-3 mg, prepare for transcutaneous pacing

8. Verapamil is classified as a(n):

    a. β-blocker

    b. natural catecholamine

    c. calcium channel blocker

    d. ventricular antidysrhythmic

9. The period of time during the cardiac cycle when cells cannot respond to a stimulus, no matter how strong, is referred to as the:

   a. vulnerable period
   b. depolarized period
   c. relative refractory period
   d. absolute refractory period

10. A 70 year old male has collapsed. A quick survey reveals the patient is pulseless and apneic. He is extremely pale and his skin is cool to the touch. CPR is initiated and a quick-look reveals the following rhythm.

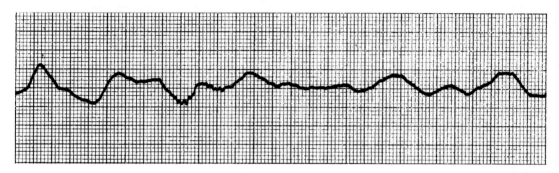

Figure 12-2

Your initial actions will include:

   a. establish IV access, intubate, and perform synchronized countershock with 50, 100, 200, 300 and 360J
   b. defibrillate immediately with 200, 200-300, 360J; resume CPR; intubate and establish IV access
   c. establish IV access, administer a 500 ml fluid challenge and prepare a dopamine drip to infuse at 5-20 μg/kg/minute
   d. intubate, establish IV access, administer 1 mg of epinephrine and 1 mg of atropine rapid IV bolus

11. Rapid, wide-QRS rhythms associated with pulselessness, shock or congestive heart failure should be presumed to be:

   a. atrial fibrillation
   b. sinus tachycardia
   c. ventricular tachycardia
   d. wide-complex tachycardia of uncertain origin

12. Select the INCORRECT statement.

    a. electric shocks produce parasympathetic discharge
    b. routine shocking of asystole cannot make the rhythm any worse
    c. in asystole, transcutaneous pacing should be considered early in the arrest situation
    d. epinephrine and atropine are administered in the management of the patient in asystole

13. In the initial resuscitation of the near-drowning victim, the rescuer should:

    a. perform the Heimlich maneuver
    b. initiate chest compressions while the victim is in the water
    c. assume cervical spine injury and support the neck in a neutral position
    d. attempt to drain water from breathing passages by administering chest compressions

14. The drug of choice in the management of torsades de pointes is:

    a. atropine
    b. procainamide
    c. isoproterenol
    d. magnesium sulfate

15. Select the INCORRECT statement regard vagal maneuvers.

    a. ice water immersion should be avoided in patients with ischemic heart disease
    b. vagal maneuvers increase parasympathetic tone and slow conduction through the AV node
    c. carotid sinus pressure should be performed carefully, with ECG monitoring, and should be avoided in older patients
    d. simultaneous, bilateral carotid massage should be attempted in the stable patient with paroxysmal supraventricular tachycardia prior to medication administration

16. When an IV lifeline is established during CPR:

    a. 5% dextrose in water is the preferred solution for use during cardiac arrest
    b. it is preferable to administer some drugs by intracardiac injection rather than IV
    c. IV medications administered by bolus injection should be followed with a 20 ml bolus of IV fluid and elevation of the extremity
    d. sites of first choice should include the external jugular or subclavian veins

17. Select the INCORRECT statement regarding the use of the bag-valve device.

   a. ideal features include a self-expanding bag, pop-off valve and transparent mask
   b. this device may be used with a mask, endotracheal tube or other invasive airway device
   c. in adults, bag-valve units usually provide less ventilatory volume than mouth-to-mouth or mouth-to-mask ventilation
   d. effective ventilation is more likely when two rescuers use the bag-valve device, one to hold the mask and one to squeeze the bag

18. Select the INCORRECT statement regarding nitroglycerin administration.

   a. nitroglycerin administration is the treatment of choice for angina pectoris
   b. nitrate-induced hypotension is best treated with administration of vasopressors, such as dopamine
   c. when administered sublingually, nitroglycerin is readily absorbed, frequently within 1-2 minutes
   d. the principal side effect of nitroglycerin administration is hypotension, which may exacerbate myocardial ischemia

A 67 year old man has walked into your Emergency Department complaining of nausea and severe chest pain radiating to his left arm and jaw. His past medical history is significant for a myocardial infarction he suffered 5 years ago. He sees his physician regularly for routine follow-up care and is presently on no medications. Your examination reveals a blood pressure of 138/76, respiratory rate of 24 and warm, diaphoretic skin. You have applied a nasal cannula at 4 liters/minute and established an IV at a keep open rate. As you attach the monitor leads, the patient tells you he feels like he is "fading". A quick glance at the monitor reveals the rhythm below. The patient is now unresponsive and pale. His blood pressure is 64/48, respirations are present but shallow at 4-6/minute. A weak, palpable pulse is present.

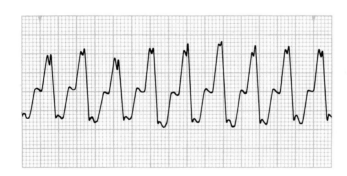

Figure 12-3 (Reproduced with permission from Huszar, RJ: *Basic dysrhythmias: interpretation and management,* 2/e, St. Louis, 1994, Mosby-Year Book, Inc.)

19. Appropriate management of this patient would include:

    a. verapamil 2.5-5.0 mg slow IV bolus
    b. countershock with 100, 200, 300 and 360J
    c. epinephrine 1 mg and atropine 1 mg rapid IV bolus
    d. lidocaine 1-1.5 mg/kg IV bolus, followed by a continuous infusion

20. Isoproterenol:

    a. is a potent, rapid-acting α-adrenergic stimulating agent
    b. is administered as a continuous infusion at a rate of 2-10 μg/min
    c. is a first-line agent used in the management of asystole due to its positive chronotropic effects
    d. is indicated in the management of pulseless electrical activity refractory to epinephrine administration

21. Advantages of central venous access over the peripheral route include:

    a. easier to learn
    b. results in fewer complications
    c. does not require interruption of CPR
    d. more rapid arrival of drugs at their sites of action

22. The preferred tidal volume for delivery of ventilations with a bag-valve device is:

    a. 5-10 ml/kg
    b. 8-10 ml/kg
    c. 10-15 ml/kg
    d. 15-20 ml/kg

23. Select the INCORRECT statement regarding the management of the cardiac arrest patient in VF.

    a. the patient's chest should be examined for the presence of a nitroglycerin patch prior to defibrillation and, if present, should be removed
    b. successive shocks are more important that adjunctive drug therapy and delays between shocks to deliver medications may be detrimental
    c. when delivering the initial "stacked" shock sequence, CPR should be performed while the defibrillator is being recharged between shocks
    d. when using conventional defibrillator paddles, the paddles should be left pressed to the chest during the delivery of the initial "stacked" shock sequence

24. You have placed an endotracheal tube and hear gurgling in the epigastrium and note an absence of chest wall movement. You have:

    a. inadvertently intubated the esophagus
    b. correctly positioned the endotracheal tube
    c. inadvertently intubated the left mainstem bronchus
    d. inadvertently intubated the right mainstem bronchus

25. Renal and mesenteric vasodilation is thought to occur with stimulation of:

    a. α-adrenergic receptors
    b. dopaminergic receptors
    c. β-1 adrenergic receptors
    d. β-2 adrenergic receptors

26. Unsynchronized countershock should be performed whenever the patient has a rapid tachycardia combined with clinical instability or whenever synchronization is delayed.

    a. true
    b. false

27. Approximately __ pounds of pressure should be applied to conventional paddles when defibrillating.

    a. 10
    b. 15
    c. 25
    d. 50

28. The correct dose for bretylium administration in VF refractory to countershock is:

    a. 5-20 μg/kg/min continuous infusion
    b. 1 mg every 3-5 minutes to a maximum dose of 0.04 mg/kg
    c. 5 mg/kg IV bolus which may be repeated with a 10 mg/kg bolus in 5 minutes
    d. 1-1.5 mg/kg repeated with 0.5-0.75 mg/kg every 5-10 minutes to a maximum dose of 3 mg/kg

29. Select the INCORRECT statement regarding endotracheal intubation.

    a. whenever possible, cricoid pressure should be applied by a second rescuer

    b. endotracheal intubation should not precede initial defibrillation attempts in VF

    c. once an endotracheal tube is in place, ventilation should be synchronized with chest compressions at a rate of 12 ventilations/minute

    d. endotracheal intubation allows adjunctive ventilatory equipment to be used more effectively and with less effort

30.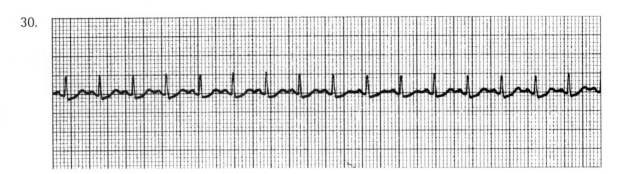

Figure 12-4

The rhythm displayed above is:

    a. sinus bradycardia

    b. sinus tachycardia

    c. ventricular tachycardia

    d. supraventricular tachycardia

31. The longest period of time for which a patient should be suctioned is:

    a. 10 seconds

    b. 30 seconds

    c. 60 seconds

    d. 90 seconds

32.

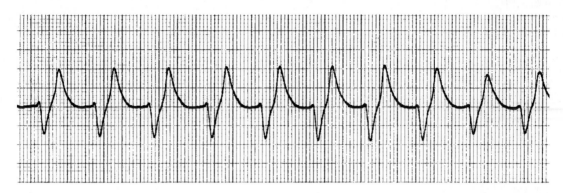

Figure 12-5

The rhythm displayed above is:

a. sinus tachycardia

b. supraventricular tachycardia

c. accelerated junctional rhythm

d. accelerated idioventricular rhythm

33. Epinephrine:

a. stimulates dopaminergic, alpha and beta receptors

b. is the first drug administered in VF, pulseless VT, asystole and pulseless electrical activity

c. dilates coronary arteries, the primary reason for administration in cardiac arrest

d. is a first-line drug in the management of the symptomatic patient with a second-degree AV block, type I

34. Morphine:

a. increases anxiety

b. decreases venous capacitance

c. is a pure β-adrenergic stimulating agent

d. decreases myocardial oxygen requirements

35. Your patient is pulseless and apneic. CPR is in progress. The cardiac monitor displays a sinus tachycardia at a rate of 110/minute. Appropriate intervention would include:

    a. intubate at once, establish an IV of normal saline or lactated Ringer's and administer a 500 ml fluid challenge

    b. intubate at once, establish an IV of 5% dextrose in water and administer adenosine 6 mg, rapid IV bolus

    c. intubate at once, establish an IV of normal saline or lactated ringer's and perform synchronized countershock with 50J

    d. intubate at once, establish an IV of 5% dextrose in water and perform unsynchronized countershock with 200J

36. In an electrical injury, the pathway of current most likely to be fatal is:

    a. foot-to-foot

    b. hand-to-hand

    c. hand-to-foot

    d. hand-to-elbow

37. Sudden death is most frequently due to which of the following dysrhythmias?

    a. asystole

    b. bradycardia

    c. ventricular fibrillation

    d. pulseless electrical activity

38. Select the INCORRECT statement regarding furosemide.

    a. furosemide may cause dehydration

    b. furosemide administration may result in diuresis

    c. furosemide's venodilating effects begin approximately 45-60 minutes after administration

    d. furosemide administration may result in hypokalemia, with subsequent cardiac dysrhythmias

39. A 46 year old male is complaining of chest pain radiating to his jaw. His blood pressure is 136/72, respiratory rate 16. The cardiac monitor displays the following rhythm:

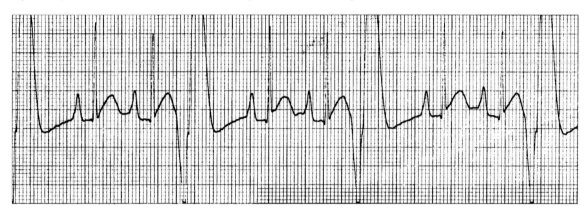

Figure 12-6

Interventions to consider in the management of this patient would include:

a. O$_2$, IV, atropine 0.5-1.0 mg IV and morphine 1-3 mg titrated to pain relief

b. O$_2$, IV, nitroglycerin, morphine if no relief from the nitroglycerin, a lidocaine bolus and maintenance infusion

c. O$_2$, IV, adenosine 6 mg rapid IV bolus, a lidocaine bolus and maintenance infusion

d. O$_2$, IV, sedation and unsynchronized countershock with 200J

40. Your patient is a 78 year old male found unresponsive, pulseless and apneic in a hospital bathroom. CPR is in progress. A quick-look reveals VT. You have delivered two of the three necessary "stacked" shocks at appropriate energy levels. The third shock will be delivered at:

a. 50J

b. 100J

c. 200J

d. 360J

A 53 year old male collapsed suddenly in the grocery store. EMTs responded to the scene and have transported the patient to your busy Emergency Department. The patient is awake, oriented and complaining of severe chest pain. He is pale and cool to the touch. Your examination reveals a blood pressure of 52/P and a respiratory rate of 18/minute. When questioned, the patient states he feels "weak and dizzy" and is nauseated. The cardiac monitor reveals the following rhythm:

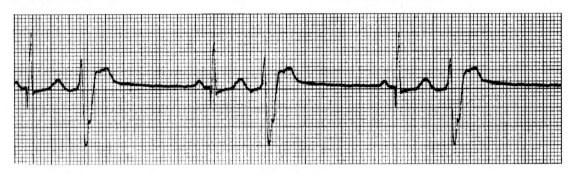

Figure 12-7

41. This rhythm is: _____.

42. Indicate your management of this patient.

A 65 year old male is complaining of "chest pressure." His past medical history is significant for an MI 4 years ago and hypertension. Medications include nitroglycerin, Cardizem and Lasix. The patient states his pain began approximately 30 minutes ago and has not been relieved by rest or the three nitro tablets he has taken thus far. His blood pressure is 144/78, respiratory rate 18. He is awake, oriented and extremely anxious. The cardiac monitor displays the following rhythm:

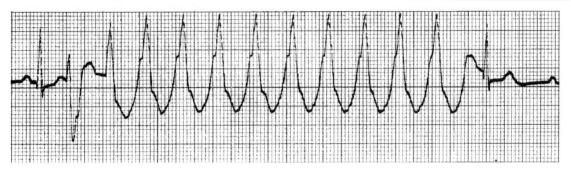

Figure 12-8

43. The rhythm shown above is: _____.

44. Indicate your management of this patient.

45. An apprehensive 76 year old female is complaining of "palpitations". She is alert and oriented and denies chest pain or difficulty breathing. Her blood pressure is 124/72, respiratory rate is 22. Your cardiac monitor shows atrial fibrillation with a rapid ventricular response of 160-190/minute. Appropriate medications to be considered for administration include:

    a. diltiazem, β-blockers, verapamil
    b. lidocaine, procainamide, bretylium
    c. isoproterenol, nitroprusside, adenosine
    d. norepinephrine, procainamide, quinidine

46. A 62 year old male is brought in to your Emergency Department by ambulance complaining of difficulty breathing. The patient is in obvious distress, gasping to breathe. His wife states he takes a "heart pill" and "water pill" for a "heart condition" but, due to their limited income, they've been unable to have his prescription refilled since he ran out of pills two weeks ago. It seems the patient has been getting progressively worse over the past couple of days and has been up walking around most of this morning trying to catch his breath. The patient's blood pressure is 170/90, pulse is 102 and irregular, respiratory rate 36 and labored. Rales are heard bilaterally on auscultation. You note the patient's feet are markedly edematous. First-line medications you will consider for use in the management of this patient include:

    a. diltiazem, propranolol and atropine
    b. verapamil, epinephrine and dopamine
    c. nitroglycerin, furosemide and morphine
    d. dopamine, norepinephrine and dobutamine

47. Which of the following statements is INCORRECT regarding second-degree AV block, type II?

    a. is usually associated with inferior wall MI and is a benign rhythm
    b. usually occurs at the level of the bundle branches, resulting in a wide QRS
    c. this rhythm may progress to complete (third-degree) AV block without warning
    d. preparations for a transvenous pacer should be made as soon as this rhythm is identified

A 67 year old male is complaining of a sudden onset of crushing chest pain which began approximately 45 minutes ago and is unrelieved with rest. He is in obvious distress, pale and profusely diaphoretic. His blood pressure is 70/44, respiratory rate 18. You have applied a nonrebreather mask and established an IV. The cardiac monitor reveals:

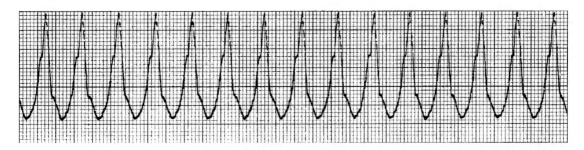

Figure 12-9

48. Considerations in the management of this patient would include:

   a. initiate CPR and defibrillate with 200, 200-300, and 360J as soon as a defibrillator is available

   b. consider medications; if no response, administer sedation, deliver a countershock with 100J and reassess

   c. consider verapamil administration; if no response, administer sedation, deliver a series of "stacked" synchronized countershocks with 50-100-200-300 and 360J and reassess

   d. administer SL nitroglycerin and, if no relief, morphine 1-3 mg IV bolus every 5 minutes until pain is relieved

49. Select the INCORRECT statement.

   a. if no IV line is in place at the time of arrest, central venous access should be attempted prior to defibrillation for VF

   b. if the femoral vein is cannulated, a long catheter must be used that extends above the diaphragm

   c. increased risks of complications are associated with placement of central lines for patients who receive thrombolytic therapy

   d. a central line may be placed in an arrest situation if spontaneous circulation does not return after initial drug administration via a peripheral vein

50. Successful completion of an ACLS provider course requires proficiency in the principles of:

   a. dysrhythmia recognition

   b. therapeutic modalities with an emphasis on algorithms

   c. basic life support, airway management and intubation

   d. all of these, according to the American Heart Association curriculum

ACLS Quick Review Study Guide

POST-TEST ANSWER SHEET

1. A   B   C   D   26. A   B   C   D

2. A   B   C   D   27. A   B   C   D

3. A   B   C   D   28. A   B   C   D

4. A   B   C   D   29. A   B   C   D

5. A   B   C   D   30. A   B   C   D

6. A   B   C   D   31. A   B   C   D

7. A   B   C   D   32. A   B   C   D

8. A   B   C   D   33. A   B   C   D

9. A   B   C   D   34. A   B   C   D

10. A   B   C   D   35. A   B   C   D

11. A   B   C   D   36. A   B   C   D

12. A   B   C   D   37. A   B   C   D

13. A   B   C   D   38. A   B   C   D

14. A   B   C   D   39. A   B   C   D

15. A   B   C   D   40. A   B   C   D

16. A   B   C   D   41. A   B   C   D

17. A   B   C   D   42. A   B   C   D

18. A   B   C   D   43. A   B   C   D

19. A   B   C   D   44. A   B   C   D

20. A   B   C   D   45. A   B   C   D

21. A   B   C   D   46. A   B   C   D

22. A   B   C   D   47. A   B   C   D

23. A   B   C   D   48. A   B   C   D

24. A   B   C   D   49. A   B   C   D

25. A   B   C   D   50. A   B   C   D

POST-TEST ANSWERS

QUESTION	ANSWER	RATIONALE	JAMA PAGE REFERENCE
1	D	The external jugular is considered a peripheral vein. The femoral, subclavian and internal jugular are central veins.	2205
2	D	Susceptibility to dysrhythmias is greatest during the early hours of infarction.	2230
3	A	Hypovolemia is the most common cause of pulseless electrical activity without measurable blood pressure.	2219
4	B	Lidocaine may be lethal if administered to a patient displaying ventricular escape rhythm (idioventricular rhythm) on the ECG.	2222
5	A	The unstable patient exhibiting sustained polymorphic ventricular tachycardia should be defibrillated with 200, 200-300 and 360 joules.	2224
6	C	The rhythm is a complete (third-degree) AV . block. The ventricular rhythm is irregular, there are more P waves than QRS's and the P waves occur regularly. There is, however, no association of the P waves to the QRS complexes.	N/A
7	D	The QRS measures <.12 sec. Administer oxygen, establish IV access and administer atropine 0.5-1.0 mg. This may be repeated every 3-5 minutes as needed to a maximum dose of 2-3 mg. *Prepare for transcutaneous pacing.*	2222
8	C	Verapamil is a calcium channel blocker.	2207
9	D	The period of time during the cardiac cycle when cells cannot respond to a stimulus, no matter how strong, is referred to as the absolute refractory period.	N/A
10	B	The rhythm is VF. Defibrillate immediately with 200, 200-300, 360J; resume CPR; intubate and establish IV access and so forth.	2217

11	C	Rapid, wide-QRS rhythms associated with pulselessness, shock or congestive heart failure should be presumed to be VT.	2205
12	B	Shocking asystole may eliminate any possibility for return of spontaneous cardiac activity.	2220
13	C	Cervical spine injury should be assumed when resuscitating the near-drowning victim, therefore the neck should be supported in a *neutral* position.	2246
14	D	The drug of choice in the management of torsades de pointes is magnesium sulfate. Isoproterenol may also be considered, *after magnesium.*	2208
15	D	Simultaneous, bilateral carotid massage should *never* be performed.	2224
16	C	IV medications administered by bolus injection should be followed with a 20 ml bolus of IV fluid and elevation of the extremity.	2205
17	A	Bag-valve devices should *NOT* have a pop-off valve because higher than normal airway pressures are often needed to ventilate the arrested patient (decreased lung compliance).	2200
18	B	Nitrate-induced hypotension usually responds promptly to fluid replacement therapy.	2210
19	B	The monitor shows a wide-complex tachycardia which should be presumed to be VT since the patient is unresponsive and hypotensive. Deliver a countershock at 100J. Reassess the patient's rhythm and pulse. If unchanged, proceed with countershocks at 200, 300 and 360J, checking pulses and rhythm in between. Due to the decreased respiratory rate and volume, intubate as soon as possible and assist ventilation with a bag-valve device.	2205

20	B	Isoproterenol should be administered by continuous infusion at a rate of 2-10 μg/min and titrated to heart rate and rhythm response. Isoproterenol is a pure β-adrenergic stimulator and is not indicated in asystole or pulseless electrical activity.	2207
21	D	Advantages of the central venous route over the peripheral route include more rapid arrival of drugs at their sites of action and successful placement even when peripheral perfusion is poor.	2205
22	C	The preferred tidal volume for delivery of ventilations with a bag-valve device is 10-15 ml/kg.	2202
23	C	When delivering the initial "stacked" shock sequence, CPR should NOT be performed while the defibrillator is being recharged between shocks.	2217
24	A	Absence of chest rise and gurgling in the epigastrium are indicative of esophageal intubation. Deflate the cuff, remove the tube and hyperventilate before reattempting intubation.	2202
25	B	Renal and mesenteric vasodilation is thought to occur with stimulation of dopaminergic receptors.	2209
26	A	True. Unsynchronized countershock should be performed whenever the patient has a rapid tachycardia combined with clinical instability or whenever synchronization seems delayed.	2226
27	C	Approximately 25 pounds of pressure should be applied equally to conventional paddles during adult defibrillation.	N/A
28	C	Bretylium is administered in VF as a 5 mg/kg IV bolus which may be repeated with 10 mg/kg in 5 minutes. The 10 mg/kg dose can be repeated every 5 minutes to a maximum dose of 30-35 mg/kg.	2218

29	C	Once an endotracheal tube is in place, ventilation should be performed *asynchronously* with chest compressions at a rate of 12 ventilations/minute.	2201
30	B	The rhythm shown is sinus tachycardia.	N/A
31	A	The longest period of time a patient should be suctioned is 10 seconds.	N/A
32	D	The rhythm shown is an accelerated idioventricular rhythm at 98 beats/minute. The rhythm is regular with a wide-QRS complex. No P waves are seen.	N/A
33	B	Epinephrine is the first drug administered in VF, pulseless VT, asystole and pulseless electrical activity. Epinephrine stimulates α and β receptors and is administered in cardiac arrest primarily due to its α-adrenergic stimulating properties. Atropine is the drug of choice in the management of symptomatic second-degree AV block, type I (associated with a bradycardic rate).	2208
34	D	Morphine decreases anxiety, increases venous capacitance, and decreases myocardial oxygen requirements. It is a narcotic analgesic.	2206
35	A	The clinical situation presented is pulseless electrical activity. Intubate at once, establish an IV of normal saline or lactated Ringer's and administer a 500 ml fluid challenge, consider the possible causes, administer epinephrine 1 mg IV bolus and so forth.	2219
36	B	The pathway of current most likely to be fatal is the hand-to-hand (transthoracic) pathway.	2248
37	C	Sudden death is most frequently due to VF.	2215
38	C	Furosemide's venodilating effects begin approximately 5 minutes after administration.	2211

39	B	The rhythm shown is a borderline sinus tachycardia with ventricular trigeminy (and R-on-T PVCs). Management of this patient should include oxygen, establishing IV access, nitroglycerin and, if no relief of pain, morphine. Due to the presence of significant ventricular ectopy seen in conjunction with the patient's presenting signs and symptoms, administer a lidocaine bolus and prepare a continuous lidocaine infusion.	2230-2231
40	D	The three "stacked" shocks are delivered at 200, 200-300, and 360J.	2217
41		The rhythm shown is a sinus bradycardia with ventricular bigeminy.	N/A
42		Administer oxygen, establish an IV and, assuming this patient's symptoms are not due to volume depletion, the drug of choice in this situation would be atropine 0.5-1.0 mg every 3-5 minutes as needed to a maximum dose of 2-3 mg. Attempt to determine the cause of the PVCs (hypokalemia, hypomagnesemia). If the patient's blood pressure improves (> 100 systolic), administer medication for relief of pain.	2221
43		The rhythm shown is a sinus rhythm with an R-on-T PVC and run of VT.	
44		Management should include administration of oxygen, IV access, morphine 1-3 mg titrated to pain relief or IV nitroglycerin may be tried, a lidocaine bolus and maintenance infusion.	2221
45	A	Medications to consider for administration to the stable patient with atrial fibrillation with a rapid ventricular response include diltiazem, β-blockers, verapamil, digoxin, procainamide, quinidine and anticoagulants.	2223
46	C	This patient is exhibiting signs of acute pulmonary edema. First-line medications include oxygen, nitroglycerin, furosemide and morphine.	2227
47	A	Second degree AV block, type II is usually associated with an anteroseptal MI.	2222

48	B	The rhythm shown is a wide-complex tachycardia. The patient is unstable as evidenced by his chest pain and accompanying hypotension. Under these circumstances, the dysrhythmia will be treated as VT. Consider medications. If no response, administer sedation and deliver a countershock with 100J and reevaluate.	2224
49	A	If no IV line is in place at the time of arrest, the antecubital or external jugular veins are the sites of first choice, *after* defibrillation for the patient in VF.	2205
50	D	Successful completion of the ACLS provider course requires proficiency in all of the areas listed, according to the American Heart Association curriculum.	2199

Index

NOTES

NOTES

NOTES

NOTES

NOTES

NOTES

NOTES

NOTES